G000321137

Vet Clinic HORSES

First published in Great Britain in 2004
by Hamlyn, a division of
Octopus Publishing Group Ltd,
2–4 Heron Quays, London E14 4JP

ISBN 0 600 60743 7

A CIP catalogue record for this book is available from the British Library

Printed and bound in Dubai

10 9 8 7 6 5 4 3 2 1

SAFETY NOTE
While the advice and information in this book is believed to be accurate, it should not be considered a replacement for professional veterinary advice. Neither the publisher nor the author can accept responsibility for any injury sustained to horse or handler while following the advice given in this book.

hamlyn

Vet Clinic HORSES

JOHN McEWEN BVMS MRCVS
ASSISTED BY JANE GLOVER-HILL BVSc MRCVS

Contents

Introduction

The purpose of this book is to help you care for your horse. It is not, however, a substitute for the equine veterinary surgeon; it is a veterinary aid for the horse owner. It can be used to help identify conditions that require urgent medical attention and lesser problems that can be treated at home. However, if you are in any doubt, always seek advice from your veterinary surgeon.

The book is designed so that you can look up the symptom or symptoms, establish the possible causes and decide on the appropriate treatment. So that you can quickly find particular problems, the book is divided into chapters covering topics such as 'The skin', 'Lameness and traumatic injury' and 'The nervous system'. The different parts of the horse have been described and illustrated in detail so that you can easily understand the many conditions from which horses can suffer. This should help you gain a greater appreciation of the problem and whether it needs immediate veterinary attention. There are also sections on first aid and on dealing with emergencies, as well as information on physiotherapy and homoeopathy.

Many problems can be avoided through good management and by correct feeding and exercise regimes, and as a horse owner you should also always be alert for the signs and symptoms that may indicate the onset of illness. If, in addition, you maintain a regular worming programme and vaccination schedule, you should be able to avoid many potential problems. The book describes these husbandry practices and includes advice on general care for all horses, from the newborn foal to the elderly horse.

Not all the conditions that might affect your horse have been included. The book deals with common conditions and the problems that are most often encountered in equine veterinary medicine. There are many more obscure conditions and exotic diseases, and as the science of veterinary medicine develops new conditions and treatments are continually being discovered. If your horse exhibits symptoms that are not covered in this book, always contact your vet for advice immediately.

Remember: if your horse is unwell or injured, seek the advice of a vet as soon as possible. This book is not a substitute for calling the vet to look at your horse. Early veterinary attention will result in the best clinical outcome in most cases, and your vet is the best person to make decisions about the treatment of your horse and will always be happy to advise you. The aim of this book is to help you understand the conditions that might arise and their possible

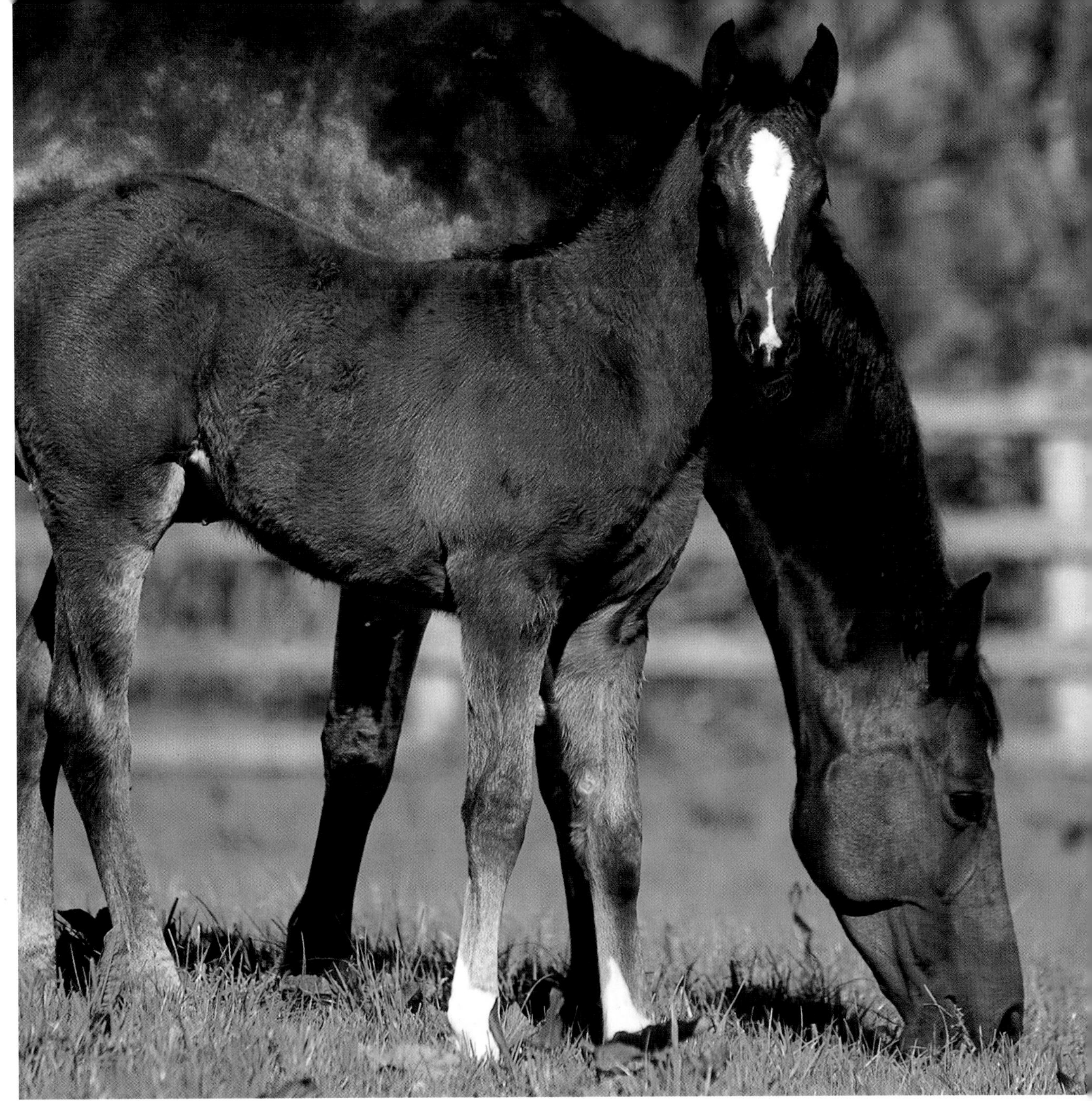

treatment and so increase the understanding between you, the horse owner, and your veterinary surgeon.

Throughout the book horses are referred to as ‘he’, unless conditions and treatments are specific to mares. In all other cases, the text applies equally to male and female horses.

Many people at my practice have helped in the production of this book, particularly the practice administrator Jeane Easterbrook, and, of course, Jane Glover-Hill. Most of all I have to thank all those horses, particularly a 33-year-old called Muffin, who have taught me so much; and my wife, Catherine, who has put up with so much.

John McEwen

Points of the horse

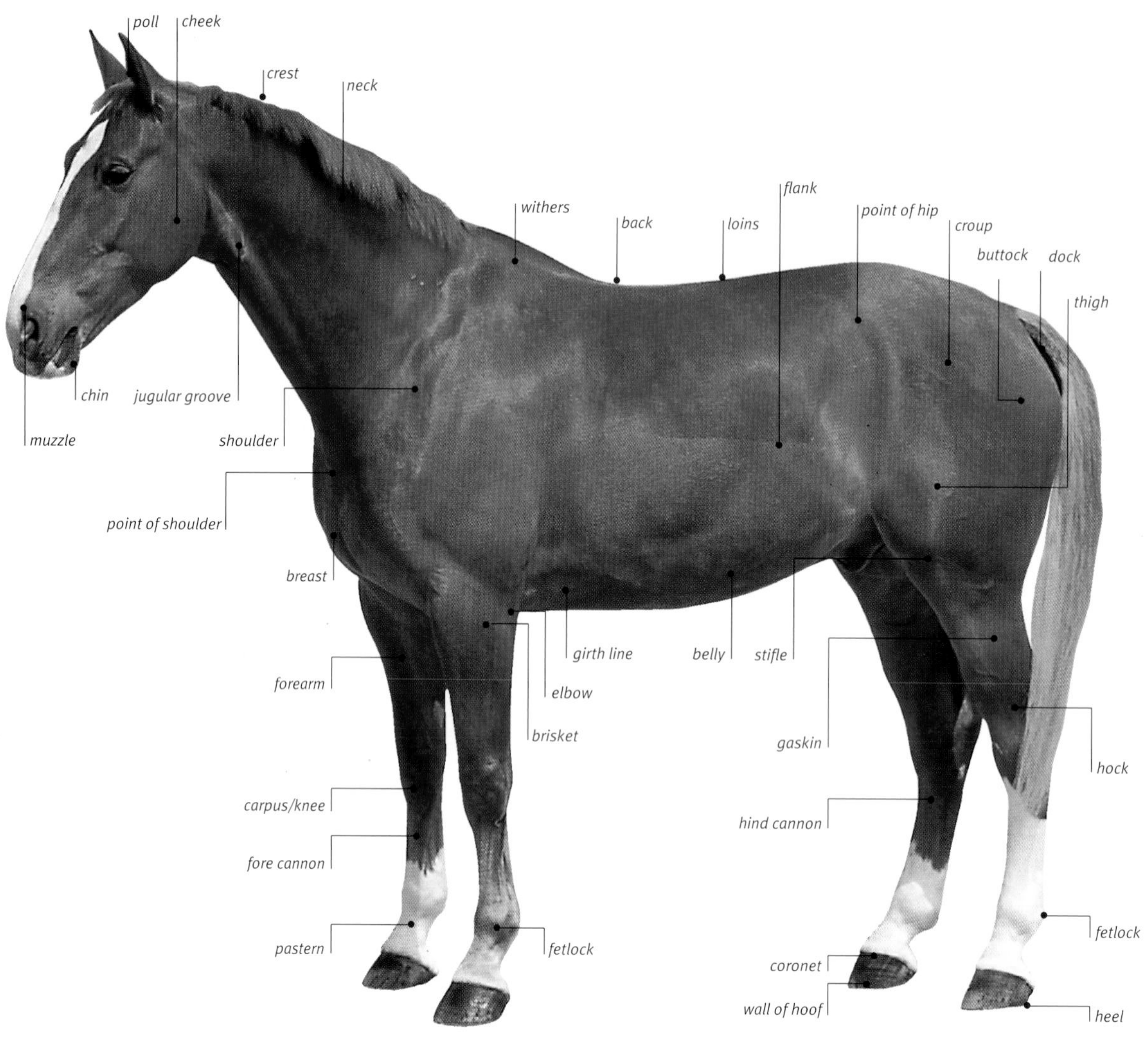

Skeleton of the horse

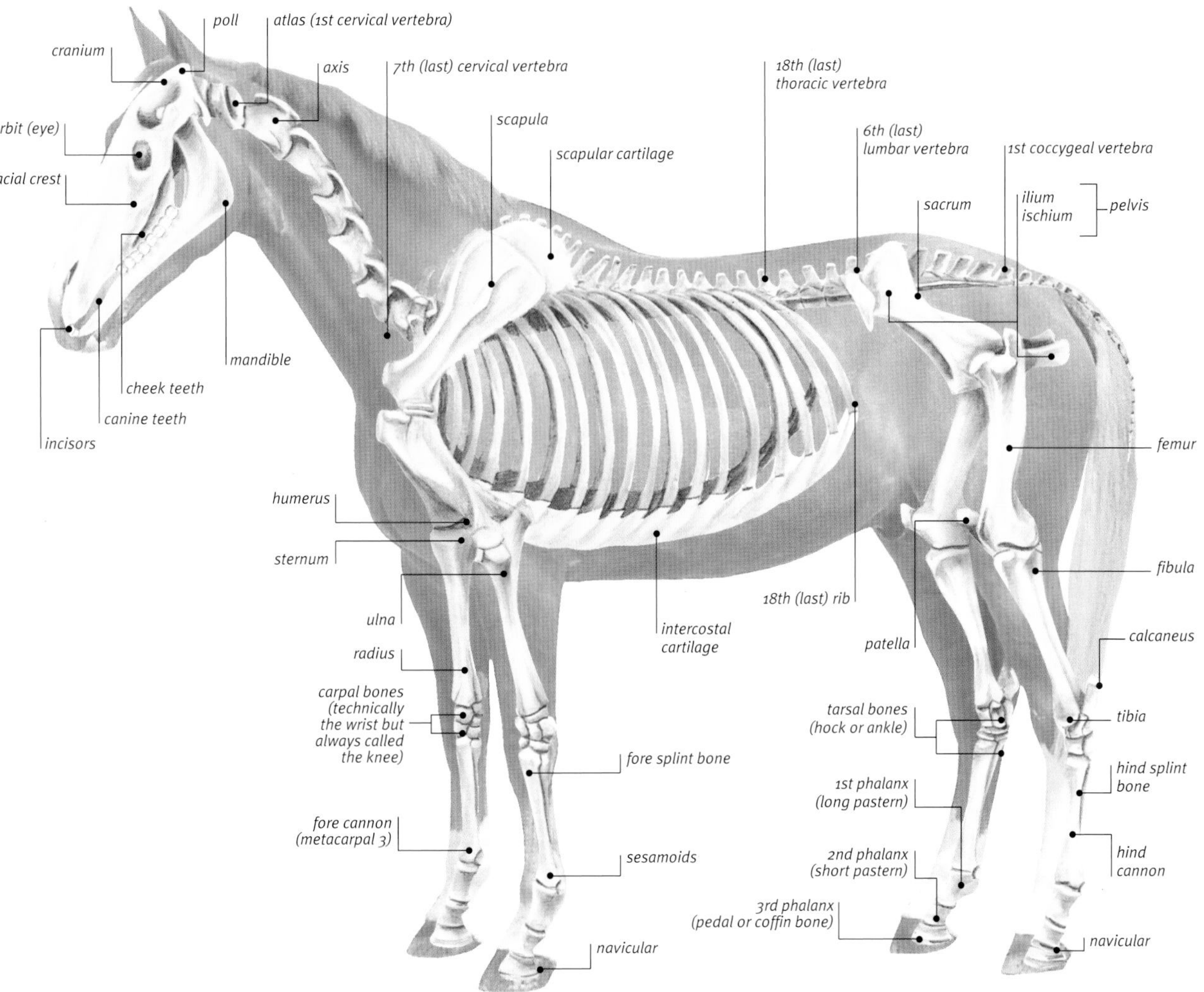

The digestive system

See Eating and drinking (pages 36–51) for ailments related to the digestive system.

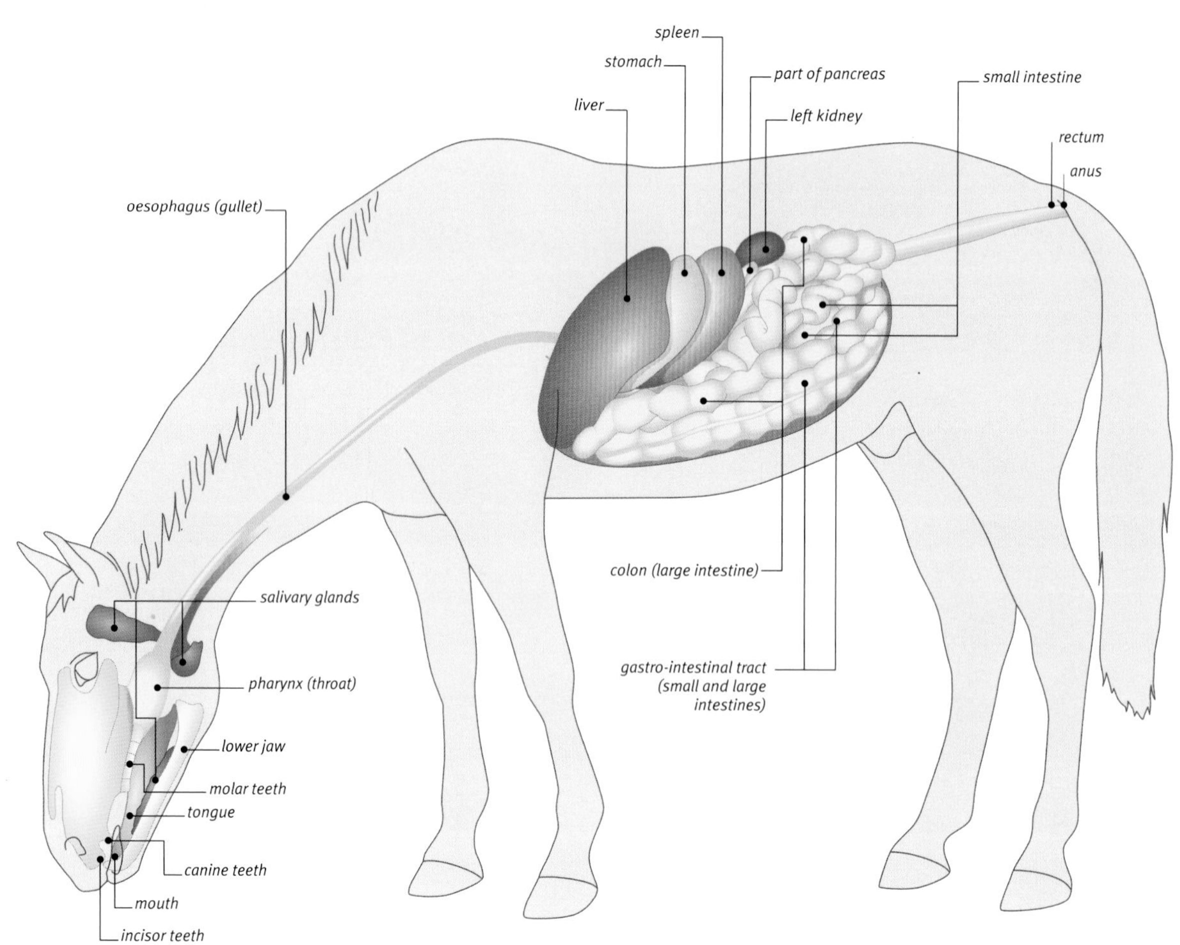

The respiratory system

See Breathing (pages 52–61) for ailments related to the respiratory system.

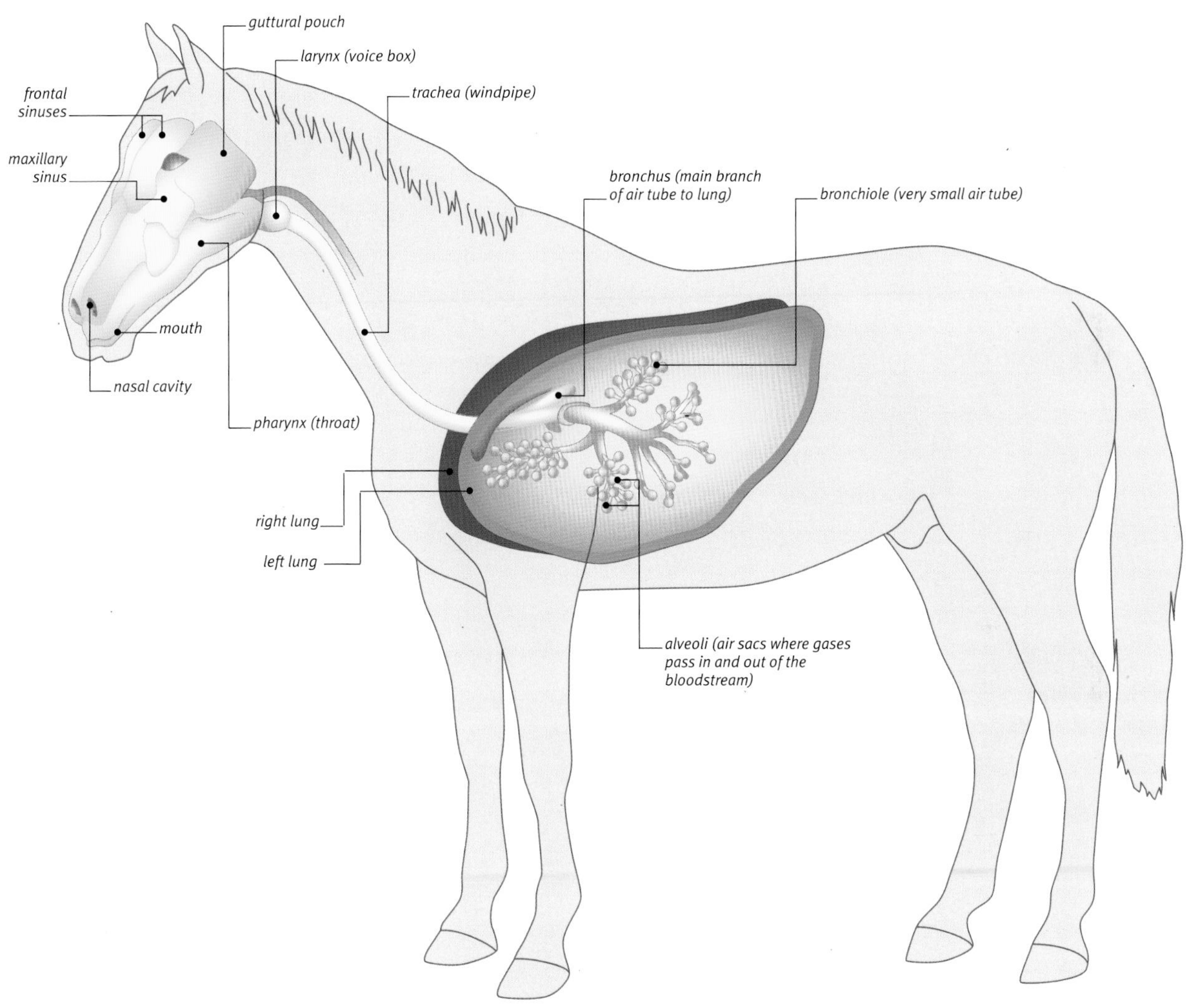

The skin

The horse's body is covered with a protective layer of skin. This is the largest organ of the horse's body and serves several functions:

- it protects the horse from the environment
- it controls body temperature by conserving heat when the horse is cold or by sweating when he is hot
- it contains pigment that protects against ultraviolet radiation from sunlight
- it is an important sensory preceptor, because horses are sensitive to touch and contact
- it secretes oils and waste products

A horse's skin is similar in many ways to that of other animals, but there are some notable differences. It contains a large number of sweat glands, and the horse sweats more easily than other animals. This specialized function is vital for maintaining a horse's core body temperature. This is important because horses are athletic animals and have a relatively large body mass to skin surface area compared with, say, dogs and cats, and may therefore have more difficulty cooling down. The sweat also contains a lot of electrolytes (minerals).

A horse's coat changes throughout the year to protect him from the extremes of both winter and summer weather. Sebaceous glands in the skin secrete oils to lubricate and waterproof the coat. The skin is also responsible for scent production, which is important because horses are social animals.

Quick-reference guide to ailments in this chapter:

For **wounds and trauma**, see pages 13–15

For **crusty and scabby skin**, see pages 16–17

For **itchy skin**, see pages 18–23

For **lumps**, see pages 24–26

For **changes in coat character**, see page 27

Wounds and scars

When skin and flesh are damaged the healing process begins, during which dead, damaged or lost tissue is replaced with the aim of returning the wounded area to its full function.

Healing

There is a difference between how well wounds above and below the knee and hock heal. The upper limbs have a good blood supply, which allows wounds to heal more quickly and more effectively. The blood supply to the lower limbs tends to be less efficient, and wounds here often have to rely on the formation of new (granulation) tissue. Unfortunately, this takes longer, produces bigger scars and often has the complication of producing excess granulation tissue.

Wounds heal in two main ways:

- **Primary intention** involves closing a wound by stitching, stapling or gluing, for example, and a small hole in the skin is quickly healed.
- **Secondary intention** refers to the healing of a wound that cannot be stitched, either because there is not enough skin to stitch or because the wound is too contaminated or old.

First aid

- Bathe the wound in a dilute solution of salty water. Do not use strong solutions or disinfectants as they will damage the remaining tissue.
- If the wound is large or deep and requires stitching, call the vet. A wound should be stitched as soon as possible and waiting for more than eight hours will delay healing and may make it impossible to stitch. If the wound is contaminated or consists of many lacerations, the vet may decide not to stitch and opt to heal the wound by secondary intention.
- Cover the wound with a sterile dressing (see pages 114–116). Gels can be applied, but generally the application of creams and oil-based products is not recommended.

Factors affecting healing

The extent of the damage and how much movement there is at the site of the wound will affect the rate at which a wound heals. Foreign material or infection will slow the healing process, as will poor blood supply, poor nutrition and reduced or elevated temperature.

Complications

- Formation of sarcoids (see page 24).
- Excessive exudates, leading to, for example, fibrinous or suppurative conditions.
- Excessive new (granulation) tissue, a common complication of leg wounds. Horses with wounds on their lower limbs should be confined to strict box rest, with adequate dressings and pressure over the wound. Wounds should be kept free from infection and antibiotics given if needed. Excessive granulation tissue may be removed surgically.

Management of large wounds

Once a wound has a healthy granulation bed, a skin graft may be necessary. This can be done in several ways. A skin graft involves the introduction of new skin cells to the wound, where they grow in the granulation tissue and allow the wound to heal from both the grafts and tissue outside the wound. Grafts help to inhibit excess granulation tissue. The grafts are normally taken from under the mane, or elsewhere on the body.

Other healing aids

- **Cold laser** helps stimulate the skin cells to heal faster and inhibits granulation tissue. The treatment must be carried out by qualified personnel.
- **Warm water therapy** will stimulate the healing cells but must be carried out gently.

JOINTS AND TENDONS

Wounds over joints or around tendons should always be checked by a vet, because an apparently small wound may actually penetrate into a joint or tendon. Joints and tendons contain synovial fluid, which lubricates the structures. It is also an ideal growth medium for bacteria. Infections in joints and tendons are potentially serious, and delay in treatment may cause irreversible damage. Wounds caused by kicks, especially if they are overlying a bony structure, should always be checked by a vet, because the force behind a kick will often cause chip fractures. If these are not spotted early and the horse given box rest, severe complications could ensue.

Photosensitivity and sunburn

Sunburn is very common in lightly pigmented horses, for example creamellos, and in coloured horses with large patches of white. A horse that has never suffered sunburn before, and then becomes very burnt for no obvious reason, is said to have become photosensitive.

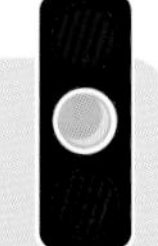

URGENCY INDICATOR

Fairly urgent, mainly to prevent further sunburn, and to help diagnose any more sinister, underlying problems.

 **COST**

Inexpensive.

Symptoms Sunburn is often restricted to light skin or hairless areas. Pink flesh and white markings on the face, the muzzle and white socks are likely to be the most sensitive areas, where there is usually inflammation and flaking of the skin. In severe cases of photosensitization, skin can peel badly. In simple sunburn, the effects are fairly superficial.

Causes The cause of sunburn is excessive exposure to ultraviolet light. Photosensitization is when normal exposure to UV light results in an unexpected and disproportional response, and a photosensitizing agent must be present in the skin for it to happen. Plants and some chemicals produce these agents. Certain liver conditions can cause secondary photosensitization, and it can also occur if the horse eats plants that are toxic to the liver. Plants of this kind, such as St John's wort, can be found in most countries but are more prevalent in some areas than others.

Owner action Remove the horse from sunlight. In mild cases, apply soothing ointments after discussion with your vet.

Treatment Protect the horse from sunlight by stabling or using hoods and rugs. Apply soothing or local anaesthetic pastes. In severe cases anti-inflammatory drugs may be required, and blood tests of liver function should be performed. Remove any plants or materials that might have triggered a photosensitive reaction.

 **DIAGNOSIS**

Made by a physical examination of the skin damage. Checking if the horse has a past history of sunburn or photosensitivity will help. The plants in the horse's pasture should also be checked in the case of photosensitivity, which can, if necessary, be confirmed by blood samples and skin biopsy.

Related conditions Greasy heel, mud fever (see page 17), bacterial dermatitis (see page 17), plant poisoning (see page 122) and fungal infections.

Prevention Beware of toxic plants and use sun block on pink-skinned areas, particularly if the horse has had problems before.

Burns and pressure lesions

Injuries to the skin caused by heat, friction, chemicals, electricity, lighting or radiation (the sun) result in the formation of burns.

Symptoms Raw, ulcerated skin or blisters.

Causes Heat or direct contact with a toxic chemical. Bandages that are too tight can also cause burns. Always put padding under a bandage (see page 116), unless it is a tail bandage, and use extra padding for pressure points such as bony prominences.

Owner action Seek veterinary advice for burns immediately. If possible, run cold water from a hose over the burn for at least 10 minutes. Do not apply any creams or dressings. If the burn is extensive, clingfilm may, with prior veterinary advice, be applied to the wound as a first aid procedure.

Seek immediate veterinary advice for chemical burns.

Treatment The treatment will depend on the cause. Always remove the cause of the injury. If necessary the horse should be given antibiotics, anti-inflammatories and analgesia to relieve pain. Severe burns may require intravenous fluid treatment and even shock therapy.

Related conditions Lymphangitis (see page 77), liver problems, and chemical and plant sensitivity.

DIAGNOSIS

Made by linking the symptoms to a prior history of exposure or bandaging.

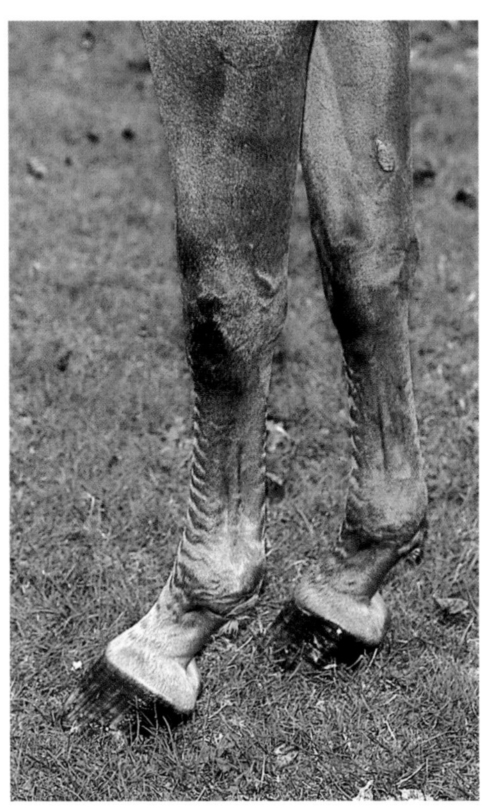

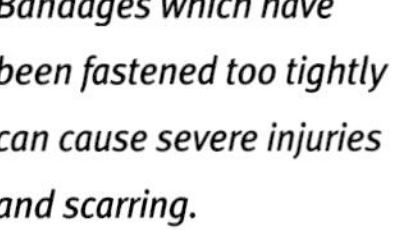

Bandages which have been fastened too tightly can cause severe injuries and scarring.

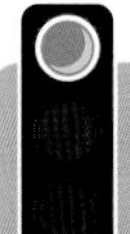

URGENCY INDICATOR

The urgency depends on the cause of injury and degree of tissue damage. Burns and pressure lesions are potentially urgent.

COST

Minor burns and pressure lesions require fairly low-cost management. As the burns become deeper, extensive wound management may be required, which becomes more expensive.
Severe burns will require intensive care, which is very expensive.

Fly strike

This occurs when flies lay their eggs in wounds or on warm, wet skin – for example, on skin contaminated with faeces or urine. The eggs then hatch into larvae, which start to feed by burrowing into any surrounding tissue.

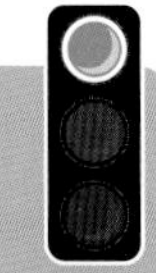

URGENCY INDICATOR

Infected wounds always need urgent attention.

COST

Low if treated early.

Symptoms Fly strike symptoms include wounds that are contaminated by fly larvae and in which active larvae are present. The wounds will not heal.

Causes Flies are attracted to discharging, infected wounds and dirty bandages. They contaminate and lay eggs in wounds. Larvae from blowfly (known as maggots in the UK) or screwfly, which are found in North and South America, live in the wounds. Screwfly larvae cause more serious secondary wound problems with extensive tissue destruction than blowfly larvae do.

Owner action Good first aid care and attention to all wounds. Liberal application of fly creams and repellents.

Treatment Any bandages should be removed and the wound should be cleaned and irrigated with saline (salt water). Visible larvae should be removed, and an insecticidal ointment or lotion containing gamma-PHC or organophosphorus (if available) should be applied to kill any larvae that remain.

DIAGNOSIS

Maggots are easily visible as small white grubs moving around in the contaminated skin.

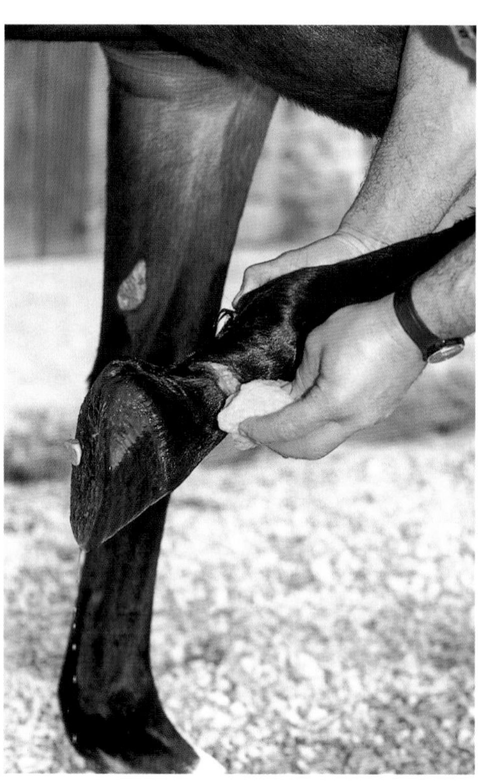

Good first aid care is vital in preventing fly strike. Wounds should be kept clean and bandages changed frequently.

Dermatitis

This condition produces crusty skin with a moist discharge, which can be seen when the crust is removed, and loss of hair. It is sometimes accompanied by swelling of the legs, caused by secondary infection.

Symptoms There are two distinct types of this kind of infection, although they overlap. The first is mud fever, which affects the lower limbs; the other is rain scald or rot, which is usually found on the horse's back and rump but may extend to other areas. It can be seen in both summer and winter but is more common in winter, particularly in wet, warm, muddy conditions. Typical initial symptoms on the lower limbs are crusty raised lesions, which are caused by bacteria, usually spreading up the limb. The heel area is particularly susceptible.

Causes An underlying skin infection or a reduction in the skin's defence mechanism. It is probably the most important and commonest skin infection and is caused by the bacterium *Dermatophilus congolensis*.

Owner action This common problem is often recurrent and difficult to avoid. If you can, reduce the horse's exposure to wet, muddy conditions and allow the legs to dry out. It can help to wash the mud off gently, using warm water and dilute chlorhexidine/poviodine. Dry the heels and apply an antibacterial ointment. This may resolve the condition, but you will need to have a good follow-up routine to protect against recurrence. This may involve using a barrier cream on clean, dry legs prior to turnout or avoiding muddy conditions altogether by stabling. Grooming equipment should be cleaned and sterilized and tack kept scrupulously clean. Rain scald also requires improved hygiene and removal from the wet. Topical anti-bacterial sprays may help to reduce the infection.

Treatment If the skin is unresponsive to first aid treatment, if the legs are swollen or if the horse is unwell, seek veterinary treatment. This may involve administration of antibiotics by injection and possibly cortico-steroid topical treatment in the form of ointment.

DIAGNOSIS

Based on the appearance of the lesions, which may be confirmed by microscopic examination of smears taken from fresh pustules and scabs.

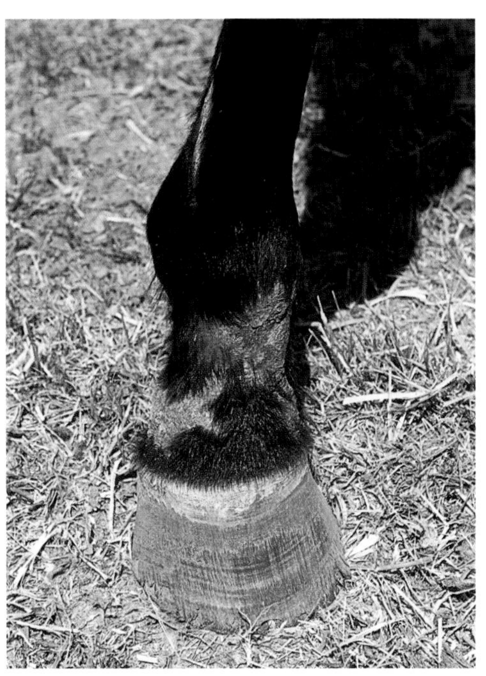

This horse is suffering from chronic mud fever of the pastern region.

Related conditions Dermatitis of bacterial origin can be confused with fungal conditions such as ringworm (see page 21) and occasionally parasitic conditions, such as lice (see page 18) or mites (see page 19).

WARNING If there is any doubt about diagnosis, or if you are dealing with a condition that you think may be mud fever but it is not responding to treatment, always seek veterinary advice.

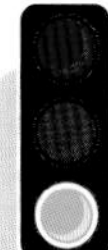

URGENCY INDICATOR

A non-urgent condition unless accompanied by illness or very swollen legs.

COST

The basic cost of treating mud fever and rain scald are likely to be low, but ongoing preventive measures will be necessary.

Lice

This is a common condition in the winter, and is often found in non-clipped or non-groomed horses. The lice either suck or bite the skin, causing itching and skin damage.

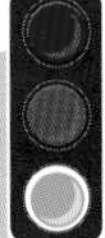

URGENCY INDICATOR

Non-urgent, but the sooner it is treated the better to prevent itching and loss of coat and condition in winter.

COST

Low, but all animals that have any contact with an infected horse must also be treated.

Symptoms Patchy hair loss on face, neck and body with generalized itching. Some degree of biting and rubbing is often seen, and the coat has a typically moth-eaten appearance. The horse may show a loss of condition. Affected horses are often very restless.

Causes There are two types of lice – biting and sucking. Sucking lice are usually found at the base of the tail and mane; biting lice are found on the lower parts of the body.

Owner action This is a common problem, and if one horse in a group has lice all the others should be checked. It is important to check for lice in horses that show a loss of condition in winter because they cause irritation, and some species suck blood and can cause anaemia. Rug hygiene is very important in these cases.

Treatment The whole body should be washed or powdered with an organo-phosphate or chlorinated hydrocarbon (where available and approved), which are very effective. pyrethroid lice powders also have some affect. All horses that have come into contact with an affected animal must also be treated. Treatment must be repeated after 10 days. Itching usually stops within a day or so of successful treatment.

Related conditions Dermatitis (see page 17), ringworm (see page 21) and some other skin conditions can look similar, so it is necessary to identify the lice before treating. If in doubt, seek veterinary advice.

DIAGNOSIS

Lice are usually visible to the naked eye and lice eggs are usually present. Use a hand-held magnifying glass to help find lice.

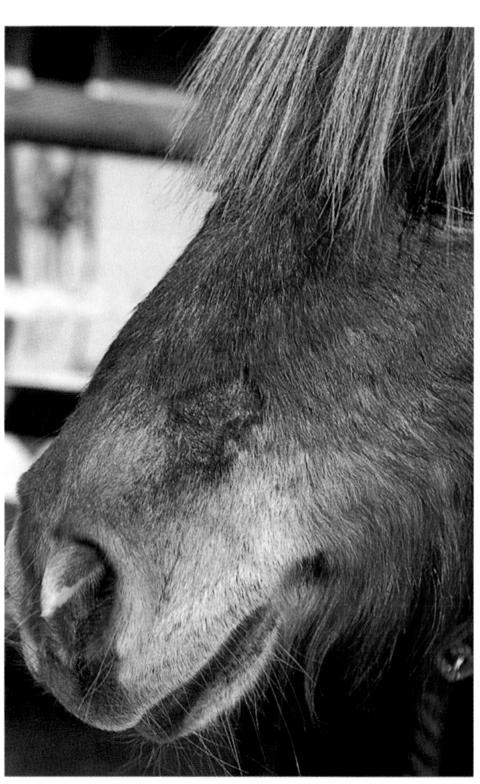

Hair loss due to lice infection is a common problem and usually affects the face and neck areas.

Mange and harvest mites

These are small skin parasites which either burrow, feed superficially or feed directly on the skin. They can cause intense itching, hair loss and skin damage.

Symptoms These conditions cause itching in varying degrees. Outward signs include leg stamping, nose rubbing, head shaking and small scabs or hair loss on the limbs, nose and, occasionally, abdomen. Severe hair loss can occur if there is repeated biting.

Causes Parasitic mites irritate the skin, and secondary bacterial infection sometimes follows. There are several types of mange mites – some burrow into the skin and others irritate the skin surface. Harvest mites and leg and tail mange tend to be seasonal problems.

The harvest mite (*Trombicula autumnalis*), which is capable of living in hay, is found on pastures and tends to infect horses' heads and limbs while they are grazing, particularly in summer and autumn.

Some mange mites, which cause chorioptic (leg and tail) mange, appear in winter, particularly in heavier and hairier breeds.

DIAGNOSIS

Finding the mites can be difficult. Surface mites are often recognized in grooming. Skin scrapings will usually confirm the presence of burrowing mites.

Owner action Because it is difficult to distinguish harvest mite infestation from mange and other forms of dermatitis, it is wise to seek veterinary advice.

Treatment The repeated use of insecticidal shampoos or powders should provide relief. Organo-phosphorus products are effective. Your veterinary surgeon may treat the conditions with an injection. Because of the infectious nature of these mites, good hygiene practice and careful stable management are important.

Related conditions Mud fever and other types of dermatitis (see page 17).

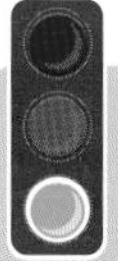

URGENCY INDICATOR

Non-urgent, but should be treated seriously and thoroughly.

COST

The cost is unlikely to be high but repeat treatment will be necessary.

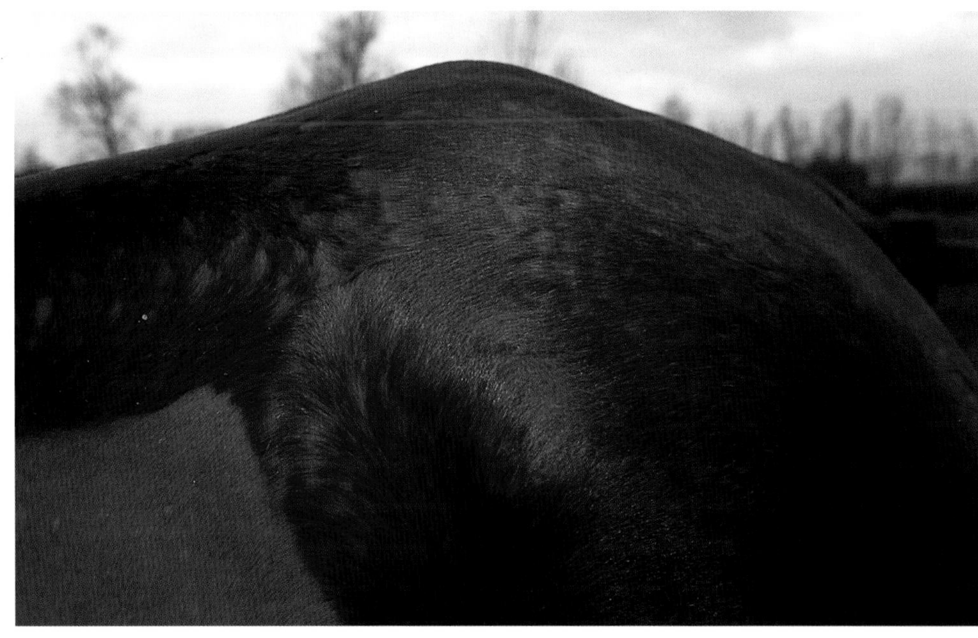

Mange causes patchy hair loss on the horse's coat, but can be difficult to diagnose due to its resemblance to other skin ailments.

Warble fly infection

The warble fly lays its eggs on the body and legs of the horse. These then hatch into larvae, which crawl up the horse's hairs and burrow through the skin into the body. They then migrate through the horse and commonly erupt through the skin in the back area.

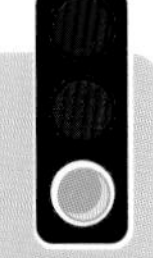

URGENCY INDICATOR

Non-urgent, but care is required because the sites of lesions can interfere with saddling and rugging.

 **COST**

Inexpensive.

Symptoms Warble fly infection usually occurs in spring and produces nodules or lumps, which are often on the horse's back. At first the lumps are firm, obvious swellings under the skin. In the later stages the actual larvae can sometimes be seen protruding from the lumps.

Causes The nodules are produced by the migrating larvae of a type of fly. The infection is primarily a disease of cattle, and the larvae do not always survive in horses and may die under the skin. Warbles are less common now that cattle are regularly treated.

Owner action Remove the horses from contact with infected cattle and treat them orally with ivermectin.

 **DIAGNOSIS**

The nodular lesions (round swellings) produced usually have breathing pores or visible larvae. The horse will normally have been in contact with infected cattle.

Treatment In addition to giving oral preparations, once the lump has burst topical treatments can be used to prevent secondary infection. Occasionally the larvae will cause an acute reaction in the horse and a secondary infection may require antibiotics.

Related conditions Eosinophilic papillomas (see page 25), abscesses (see page 26), fly bites and saddle sores.

Pinworm infestation

Pinworms are small worms that live in the horse's intestine and cause intense itching of the tail area when they lay their eggs.

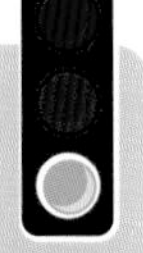

URGENCY INDICATOR

Early treatment is advisable to prevent spread to other horses.

 **COST**

Inexpensive.

Symptoms Excessive tail rubbing, with sores at the base of the tail created by the rubbing.

Causes A worm, *Oxyuris equi,* that lives in the last part of the bowel and in the rectum is the culprit. The adult worms lay eggs around the rectum.

Owner action Regular worming and good stable hygiene, with local treatment including washing the area with soap and water to remove the eggs, and in some cases treating the secondary sores with soothing ointments.

Treatment See owner action.

 **DIAGNOSIS**

Based on the intense itching around the anus, and greyish-yellow egg masses on the perineal skin. The larger white female worms may be seen in the faeces.

Related conditions Lice (see page 18), mites (see page 19), dermatitis (see page 17) and sweet itch (see page 23).

Ringworm

Ringworm is a common fungal infection of the horse's skin (epidermis and hair follicles). It is more common in the winter months, and is highly infectious.

Symptoms Loss of hair, usually initially in patches that may join together into larger areas, sometimes with itching and secondary infection. In the initial stages the hairs in some areas may be erect. Within 12 days of initial infection the hairs can be easily plucked out of the site. Common areas of infection are the horse's girth, shoulders and chest, resulting from contamination from girth and riding boots. Generalized infection is common in young horses.

Causes Ringworm is an infectious fungus. There are two types, *Tricophyton* and *Microsporum* spp.

Owner action Separate and isolate both horse and tack from others, remembering that indirect contact via gateposts, stable doors and feed buckets can transfer infection. Sterilize all tack and premises with antifungal agents.

Treatment This involves fungicidal treatment of the horse and sporadic treatment for the surrounding environment as discussed above. The infected areas of the horse should be clipped, taking care to disinfect the clippers at regular intervals.

Related conditions Dermatitis (see page 17), lice (see page 18) and mites (see page 19).

Prevention Good stable hygiene and the isolation of early cases will reduce the possibility of outbreaks.

Note Horses that have been in contact with an infected animal should also be washed with a fungicide. Washing twice-weekly with a shampoo containing 2 per cent miconazole and 2 per cent chlorhexidine can reduce cross-infection and so limit further outbreaks. Spot treatments may be of some use, but their value is limited because of the speed with which ringworm spreads. Topical treatments such as natamycin are effective. Oral preparations containing griseofulvin administered daily over long periods on veterinary advice can also be useful but should not be used alone.

DIAGNOSIS

Based on clinical signs and history of contact with infectious horses. Microscopic inspection of hair from fresh lesions and culturing of hair in special media will confirm the diagnosis.

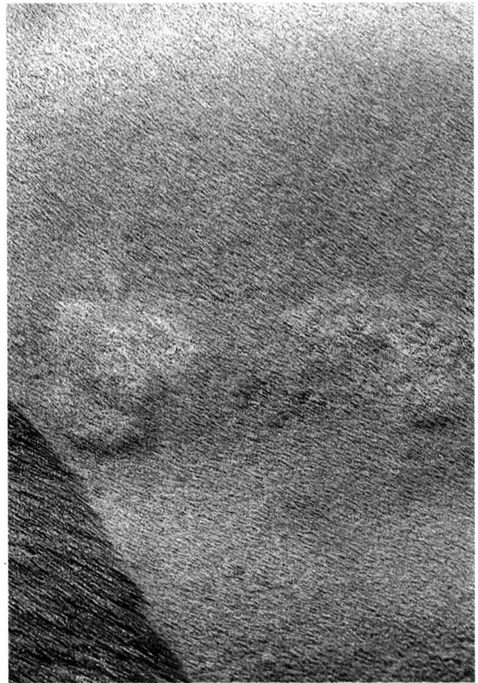

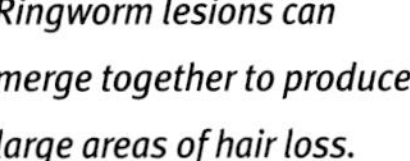

Ringworm lesions can merge together to produce large areas of hair loss.

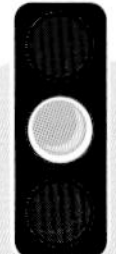

URGENCY INDICATOR

Early treatment is necessary to prevent rapid spread on the patient and to other horses.

COST

Initial washes and oral preparations are not too expensive, but costs add up if treatment needs to be carried out over a long period due to re-infection.

Insect and snake bites

A wide number of insects bite horses. Snake bites are less common, but are usually found on the muzzle and legs, and often appear as two small visible holes caused by the snake's fangs.

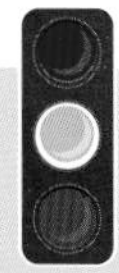

URGENCY INDICATOR

Depends on the severity of the reaction to the sting and the number of stings. All animals that have been stung should be kept under close observation for an hour or two after the sting in case a more severe reaction develops. Snake bites should always receive immediate veterinary attention and in areas where snakes are common, snake bites should always be considered as possible causes of swelling around the lower limbs and on the head and nose.

COST

Low, because minor bites and stings do not usually have serious consequences.

Symptoms A horse's reaction to a bite depends to some degree on the type of insect and the area of skin bitten, but usually there is an initial inflammatory response, which includes swelling and sometimes pain and irritation. There may also be secondary reactions, including infection with scabbing and discharge. More severe reactions may occur, including swelling of larger areas of the body, particularly the head, face and limbs. Severe secondary symptoms include respiratory distress, unsteadiness of limbs and, on rare occasions, collapse and death. Multiple stings can cause severe reaction and shock and, occasionally, death.

Causes Bites from horse, stable, buffalo, horn, black and louse flies as well as mosquitoes, bees, wasps and biting spiders (depending on the part of the world) and tick infestation. Biting insects tend to produce localized reactions and some degree of worry and agitation, while toxins injected by stinging insects can cause more severe reactions.

Owner action Check the bitten areas and try to identify the biting insect. Assess the degree of distress that the horse is in and telephone for veterinary advice. The need for veterinary attention depends on the degree of reaction to the bite or sting, but if swelling is rapidly increasing and the horse is in distress, urgent veterinary attention should be sought. If the swelling is small and localized and has obviously been present for some time, the condition is usually not urgent.

First aid treatment should include cleaning the area with cold water containing a pinch of salt or a small amount of disinfectant and removing the horse from the possibility of any more bites.

Treatment This depends on the severity of the condition and type of insect involved. Treatments can include mild, topical, anti-inflammatory preparations, injections to reduce reaction, antibiotics and corticosteroidal creams. It is helpful to identify the insect concerned because wasps and biting spiders tend to have alkaline bites, whereas bee stings are acid: the application of vinegar to one and bicarbonate solution to the other may reduce the immediate painful effects.

DIAGNOSIS

This depends on the history of the bite and the horse's reaction.

Prevention Careful disposal of manure, control of vegetation around stable areas, and the use of insect repellents in stables and around yards, topical insecticidal preparations on the horse and mesh to stop insects getting into stables will all help. Insect traps and repellent strips can also be effective.

Sweet itch

Sweet itch is a hypersensitivity or allergy to midge bites. The condition is rare in foals and young horses and is usually seen from the age of four onwards. The symptoms are seasonal, and the condition usually worsens with age.

Symptoms A continual itch, which is usually worse in the early mornings and evenings, when the midges are flying. The irritation can lead to weight loss. The affected sites are usually at the base of the tail and on the neck, mane, head and back. These areas will usually have been rubbed, so you see bald or raw patches, crusty scabs and loss of hair in the mane and tail. In more chronic cases there is usually a thickening of the skin, which often causes ridges, particularly in the mane and sometimes in the tail.

Causes Hypersensitivity to midge bites.

Owner action The best way to control the condition is to reduce the chance of the horse coming into contact with midges. Act early, and if your horse has had the problem before take preventative action. Use fly control and fly repellent whenever possible.

Treatment If the condition is serious it needs to be treated topically (on the skin) and, in some cases, systemically (orally or with injections) in order to control it. Antihistamines and cortico-steroids may be necessary and must be coupled with fly repellent and fly control to complete the treatment.

Topical fly repellent in the form of sprays and lotions, such as benzyl benzoate, citronella oil, pyrethrins and synthetic pyrethroids can help when applied to the rugs, head, mane, backs and tails of individual horses. Attaching cattle fly ear-tags to headcollars and rugs has proved successful in some cases. Rugs and protective head nets have also produced good results; rugs are now marketed specifically for this purpose.

It is most important to protect the horse from midges. Stabling while the midges are at their worst, particularly in early mornings and from afternoon to dusk, with rugs and hoods or in insect-proof stabling helps to prevent the problem. It is also useful to have good hygiene around the stables and to make sure that the muck heap is not close to where the horse is kept or that the muck is regularly disposed of a long way from the stable area.

Related conditions Lice (see page 18), pinworm (see page 20), other biting flies, insect bites (see page 22) and chemical irritation.

DIAGNOSIS

Based on evidence of the symptoms described, as well as the seasonal characteristics. Other skin parasites should be eliminated as the cause but it is usually fairly easy to distinguish.

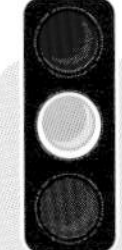

URGENCY INDICATOR

Non-urgent, but results are much more likely to be successful if treatment is started promptly.

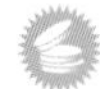

COST

Relatively low, but ongoing preventive measures can be costly.

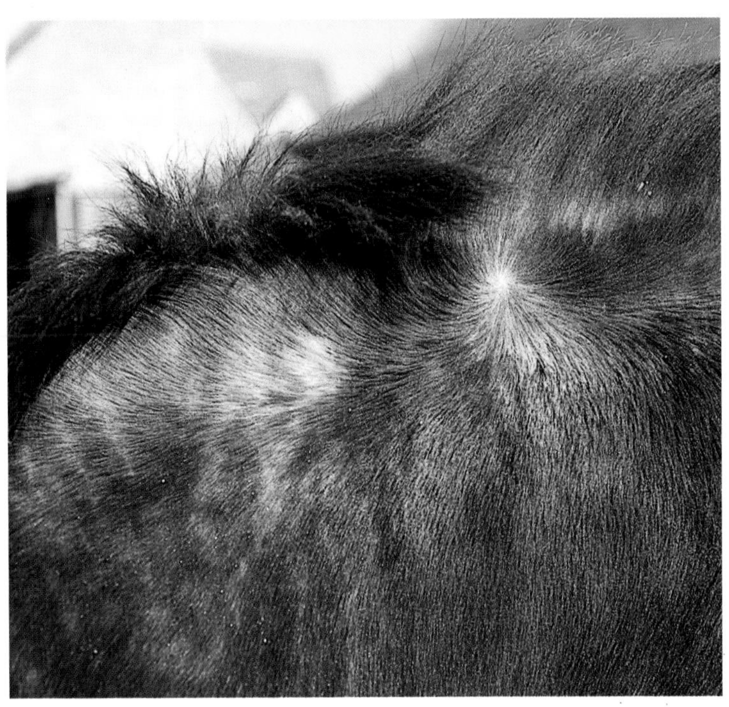

The neck and mane is a common site of sweet itch on the horse.

Skin tumours

Horses can suffer from several different types of skin tumour. Veterinary help should always be sought to identify the type of tumour and advise on appropriate treatment.

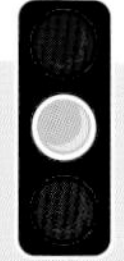

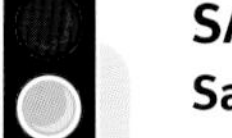

URGENCY INDICATOR

Early diagnosis and treatment is often beneficial.

COST

Expensive. The initial treatment can be costly (general anaesthesia may be required), and this is frequently combined with follow-up treatments.

SARCOID TUMOURS

Sarcoid tumours are probably the most common skin tumours found in horses. They occur in many different forms, and veterinary diagnosis is always necessary. A 'less severe form' can rapidly progress to a more aggressive tumour if left untreated.

Symptoms The tumours can be found anywhere on the horse's body, but the most common sites are around the hindquarters, on the belly, inside the thighs and on the head, face and neck. The tumours can appear as thickened flaky skin, as round, nodular masses or raw ulcerative lumps. They are sometimes joined to the body by pedicles (stem-like strips of tissue).

Causes At present there is controversy over the cause of this type of tumour, but they are probably viral in origin and are more common in younger horses.

Owner action The diagnosis must be confirmed by a veterinarian, and treatment will depend on the type and site of the tumour.

DIAGNOSIS

Some sarcoid tumours may be visibly diagnosed by a vet, but if unsure a biopsy should be taken and sent for laboratory analysis.

Treatment Many treatments can be used for sarcoids, some of which are not conventional, and they may have to be used in combination. Surgical methods include ligation (removal by tying) of the pedunculated tumour or surgical excision. However, there tends to be a high rate of recurrence.

Other courses of action include cryosurgery, where the tumour tissue is frozen, dies and drops off; and electro-cautery and laser incision, where the tumour is cut out. There may also be local topical medication with a cytotoxic or a chemotherapeutic preparation, or the use of vaccines (autogenous or BCG locally).

Related conditions Melanoma (see below), abscesses (see page 26), warble fly (see page 20) and other skin tumours.

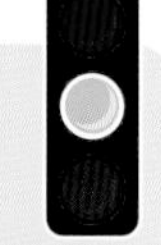

URGENCY INDICATOR

Non-urgent, unless the tumour is rapidly growing and spreading, but always seek veterinary advice.

COST

Expensive if extensive treatment is necessary.

MELANOMAS

Melanomas are tumours of the pigment cells. They are benign (non-invasive) tumours but may cause problems because of their bulk and the space they occupy. A rare form of melanosarcoma is rapidly invasive to other organs, such as the liver and kidney.

Symptoms These tumours are usually visible as hard, spherical nodules of variable size. They are usually slow growing and are commonly found around the rectum, vulva and tail areas, although they can occur anywhere on the body. Melanomas can ulcerate and produce a thick, black, tarry discharge or can sometimes join together to form thick groups of nodules.

DIAGNOSIS

Melanoma is usually diagnosed by its characteristic appearance and location. In doubtful cases a needle biopsy, which produces black pigmented material, is usually enough to confirm diagnosis. Histopathology is rarely required, but requires the complete removal of the tumour.

Causes As with most tumours, a cause is not yet known, but they are very common in aged grey horses.

Owner action Because melanomas only grow slowly the owner need take no urgent action.

However, it is sensible for the vet to confirm the diagnosis and advise on treatment.

Treatment Small, single tumours can be removed surgically. Cryosurgery can be used in more complicated cases but rarely cures the problem. Other treatment involves the injection of cystoplatin into small tumours, and there is some reported usage of cimetidine (an anti-ulcer drug) given orally for actively growing tumours. In many cases – particularly older, grey horses – melanomas are best left untreated, although veterinary advice should always be sought in case more aggressive melanosarcomas develop.

Related conditions Sarcoids (see opposite), abscesses (see page 26), warble fly (see page 20) and other rare skin tumours.

EOSINOPHILIC PAPILLOMAS

These are one of the most common nodular skin conditions in horses. They are possibly the result of local hypersensitivity to insect bites, although in some cases there is no insect contact. Treatment is only necessary if there is secondary infection.

PAPILLOMAS

Papillomas are common warts caused by a virus. In young horses they are often found in large numbers around the muzzle and face.

Symptoms Papillomas appear as pink or grey warts, particularly on the muzzle and around the eyes and face. Although occasionally seen in older horses, this condition usually affects horses up to about four years of age. It is moderately contagious by direct and indirect contact between horses that graze together and is sometimes known as grass warts.

Causes This is a viral skin condition of the papillomas group and can be transmitted by black flies or by direct or indirect contact.

Owner action A veterinary surgeon should confirm the diagnosis. It may be sensible to isolate the infected horse until the problem is resolved to prevent it from spreading.

Treatment Treatment is not usually required because papillomas often disappear spontaneously after three or four months. If treatment is necessary autogenous vaccines may be tried, although there is some doubt about their efficacy. Surgical removal may be necessary in sites around the eyes, and cryosurgery can be used to remove unsightly warts. There is little or no spontaneous regression in older horses.

 **DIAGNOSIS**

The appearance described left is usually enough to make a diagnosis in a young horse.
If necessary, a biopsy or histopathology can be carried out.

Related conditions Sarcoids (see opposite), other skin tumours.

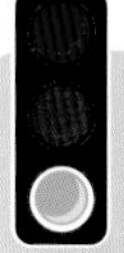

URGENCY INDICATOR

Non-urgent.

 **COST**

Treatment is not usually required.

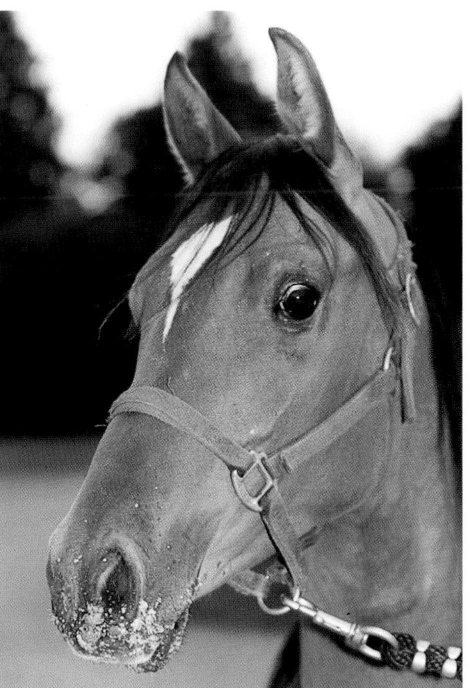

Multiple papillomatous warts are visible here around the muzzle of a young horse.

Abscesses

Abscesses are localized swellings, usually a collection of pus in a cavity, which may occur in any part of the body. They can be caused by foreign bodies, infections or trauma.

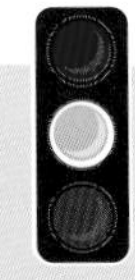

URGENCY INDICATOR

Rarely an extreme emergency, but they should receive veterinary attention without undue delay because of the risk of infection and tetanus.

COST

Unlikely to be very high, although it will depend on the site and extent of the abscess. Any surgical procedures can be performed under local anaesthetic or sedation.

Symptoms Swellings, sometimes small, sometimes large, which may come to a head and discharge pus. They may be infected or sterile and may come up suddenly or be relatively slow to develop.

Causes Abscesses are caused by localized infection or by tissue destruction. The infection sometimes gains access through a wound or puncture of the skin, but they are also sometimes caused by blood-borne infections. Parasites may cause abscesses, and sterile abscesses usually develop in response to non-infectious tissue damage.

Owner action It is often helpful to apply a hot cloth in the form of a poultice to the abscess. Veterinary attention will be required to treat the underlying infection with drainage and antibiotics and, particularly, to administer anti-tetanus treatment, because most abscesses are caused by penetrations and wounds.

Treatment Treatment will depend on the nature and site of the abscess. The most common treatment is to create good drainage and to use antibiotic therapy to treat any underlying infection, combined with poultice and tetanus therapy.

It is important to make sure that any purulent discharge from the abscess has not damaged the surrounding skin areas, and the application of petroleum jelly or a similar product to the surrounding areas will help prevent this.

Related conditions Haematoma (severe bruising), swelling from physical injury, solar abscess (see page 73) and strangles (see page 55).

DIAGNOSIS

Initially made on the basis of a hot, painful swelling of the skin. The site should be inspected for possible associated wounds or penetrations and for other smaller swellings elsewhere. The abscess may be swabbed to rule out strangles.

Cushing's disease

This is a condition caused by an overactive adrenal gland. In the horse, this is secondary to an overactive pituitary gland which stimulates the adrenal gland, and is usually associated with a pituitary tumour. It is common in older horses, and causes characteristic coat changes.

Symptoms Failure to lose coat and a typically curly coat, which is often put down to old age. Apart from being curly and not shedding, the coat often feels sweaty and sticky, and the horse sometimes suffers from secondary infections. Wounds that won't heal should make you suspicious. Look out for unresponsive and recurrent laminitis, and excessive drinking and urinating. The horse may also suffer from weight loss and lack resistance to infection.

Cause This is caused by a common tumour in the brain. The tumours are small, and the disease is usually seen in horses over 12 years old. The size of tumour is not directly related to the physiological effects on the horse.

Owner action If the older horse begins not to shed his coat in summer and the nature of the coat changes, or if you notice your horse is drinking and urinating more, seek veterinary advice.

DIAGNOSIS

The symptoms described are fairly characteristic. Blood sugar levels can also be abnormal. Blood tests, such as ACTH stimulation tests and dexamethasone suppression tests, may be carried out. These enable the output from the adrenal gland to be monitored, and an overactive adrenal gland to be diagnosed.

Treatment Treatment involves careful management. Various medications have been used, but you should discuss the value of medical treatments with your vet.

Related conditions Diabetes, kidney failure, sweating problems and other causes of laminitis (see page 74) and immune suppression.

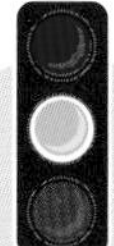

URGENCY INDICATOR

Urgent if laminitis is involved, otherwise the condition comes on gradually.

COST

Expensive therapy can prolong life by several years but must be sustained.

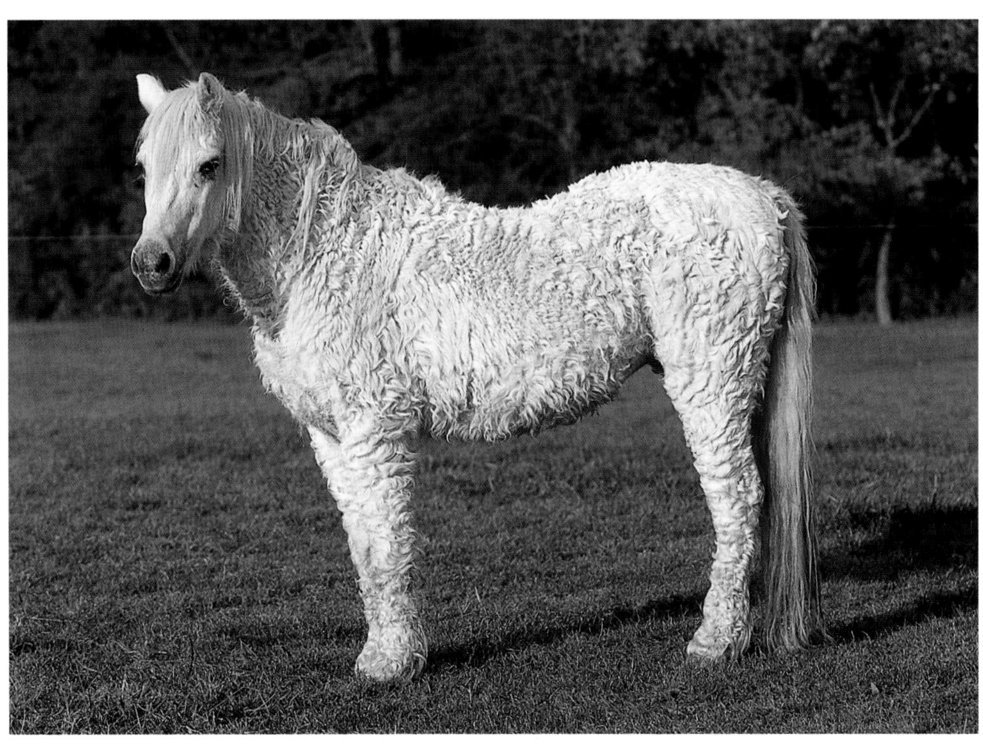

The very curly coat on this old pony is a classic indicator of Cushing's disease.

Eyes and ears

The eyes and ears of the horse are his most important sensory organs. They are highly developed in order to help the horse survive in the wild, giving wide-angle vision and a rapid response to noises that may indicate a threat.

THE EYE

The horse's eye is a complex, vital organ that has evolved to aid his survival in the wild. The eyeball or globe consists of three layers: the outer layer, which includes the cornea; the middle layer, which contains the iris; and the inner layer, which contains the retina. The transparent part of the eyeball, the cornea, allows the horse to see out, and the iris and the pupil are visible through it. The middle layer contains ligaments holding the lens, which focuses light on the retina, which in turn contains light-sensitive cells.

A horse needs good peripheral vision, and any injury or damage to the eye must receive immediate veterinary attention. **Warning! Never try to treat any eye problems yourself – always seek veterinary advice.**

THE EAR

The horse's ear has three main parts: the eardrum, which changes sounds to vibrations; the middle ear, which contains the ossicles that transmit the vibrations from the eardrum to the inner ear; and the inner ear, where the vibrations are translated into electrical signals and transmitted to the brain, which interprets the sound.

Horses have specialized ears. Each ear can independently swivel through 180 degrees or be laid back to shut out sound. This amazing mobility is achieved by 16 muscles attached to the base of the pinna, the external, visible ear flap (in contrast, a human has only three such muscles).

Horses use their ears to signal their emotional state and intent as well as to protect against over-loud sounds and focus directional sounds. They are able to hear higher pitched tones than humans – at 25kHz and above they can hear sounds almost an octave higher than we can. In the middle range the horse is capable of hearing small differences in tone, and, as all horse owners know, they are very sound-sensitive animals.

Quick-reference guide to ailments in this chapter:

For **a red, painful eye**, see pages 29–31

For **problems of the eyelid**, see page 32

For **loss of vision**, see page 33

For **swellings in or around the eye**, see page 34

For **problems of the outer ear**, see page 35

Conjunctivitis

Inflammation of the membrane on the inner eyelid and over the eyeball, or third eyelid, causes reddened eyes and may affect one or both eyes. It may be acute (appears rapidly) or chronic (lasts a long time and resists treatment).

Symptoms Reddened eye with discharge and increased tear production, half-closed eyes and occasional rubbing of the eyes.

Causes The condition can be caused by fly worry, allergies, infections (bacterial, viral or fungal) or physical damage (scratches or foreign bodies, such as grass seeds). The most common cause is bacterial infection.

Owner action Check the eyes regularly when you are grooming or feeding your horse. Carefully examine the eye if any discharge or swelling is noted. The eye may be gently bathed with a little cotton wool soaked in warm water. Never put cotton wool into the eye itself. Instead, pass the cotton wool over the eyelids and squeeze slightly so the water washes gently over the eye. Do not try to remove foreign bodies from the eye using tweezers (forceps) or cotton wool buds, because sudden movement caused by the sensitivity of the eye may well result in further damage.

Treatment Treatment depends on the cause of the problem. The vet may prescribe antibiotics, in the form of ointment or drops, and anti-inflammatory drugs, to be applied topically, orally or by injection, depending on the severity of the condition. With all eye conditions, treatment must be regular with frequent treatment many times a day. Problems may arise as horses can sometimes resent having ointment or drops put in their eyes. However, most cases respond quickly to a course of antibiotics.

Related conditions Periodic ophthalmia (see page 30), corneal ulceration (see page 31), problems of the eyelid (see page 32), cataracts (see page 33) and tumours of the eye (see page 34).

DIAGNOSIS

Made from the symptoms of eye discharge and inflammation. Bacteriology and sensitivity tests can be carried out on the discharge, and fluorescence staining (when a weak solution of stain is dropped into the eye, highlighting any damage) is often done to show any ulceration of the cornea. It can also reveal if there is any obstruction to the lasso lacrimal (tear) duct (the eye's drainage system).

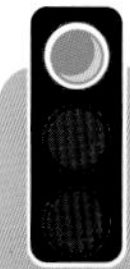

URGENCY INDICATOR

Urgent, especially if there are complications, such as foreign bodies in the eye.

COST

Relatively low in simple cases.

THE EYE

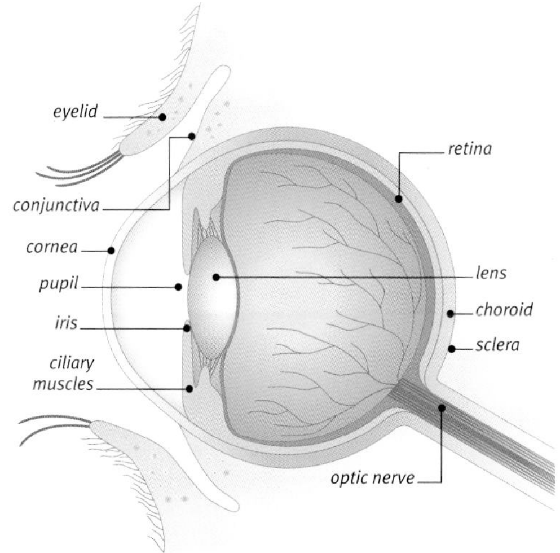

A cross-section of the horse's eye.

Periodic ophthalmia

Periodic ophthalmia or recurrent uveitis (moon blindness) is the most common disease of the iris (uveal tract). Together with eye tumours and ulcers, it is one of the most common causes of blindness in horses.

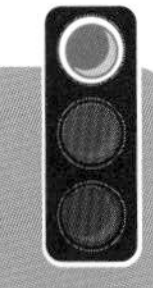

URGENCY INDICATOR

Urgent – the earlier the treatment, the better the end result.

COST

Not a particularly expensive condition to treat but there will be ongoing expense because of the recurrent nature of the disease.

Symptoms The iris is in spasm and the affected eye will make excessive tears, which often run down the face. The eyelid will often be half-closed and the eye itself will appear cloudy. Bright light will cause pain, so the horse will avoid it if at all possible. The eye may also appear to be cloudy or white.

Causes In most cases of periodic ophthalmia, the causes cannot be determined. There have, however, been suggestions of a number of causes, including a response to traumatic or immune-mediated inflammations, viral inflammations, bacterial inflammations, parasites or vitamin deficiencies. Treating the symptoms is effective, at least in the short term.

Owner action Urgent, because if an eye is not treated promptly then irreversible damage, affecting sight, can occur. If in doubt, seek veterinary advice.

Treatment Treatment aims to reduce inflammation and changes within the eye. It will involve the use of cortico-steroids and non-steroidal anti-inflammatory drugs to reduce pain and inflammation. The vet will probably recommend eye drops to dilate the pupil, which helps to counteract the pain from the spasm of the iris.

Related conditions Acute conjunctivitis (see page 29), haematoma (severe bruising), corneal ulceration (see page 31) and trauma.

WARNING This condition has a high rate of recurrence, and observation and early treatment will be necessary in future.

DIAGNOSIS

Diagnosis depends upon the symptoms of intense eye pain and excessive tear production and discharge, coupled with photophobia (pain in bright lights) and clouding of the eye (corneal oedema). The most consistent symptom is constriction of the pupil so careful examination of the iris should be made.

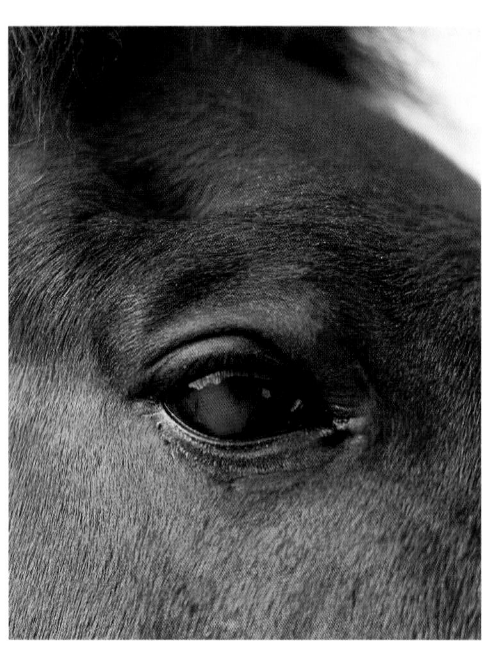

Periodic ophthalmia, or moon blindness, requires urgent treatment to prevent irreversible damage.

Corneal ulceration

Ulcers occur on the cornea when trauma, foreign bodies or infection damage and roughen the surface, which is usually smooth.

Symptoms Usual signs are blinking, discomfort, increased discharge from the eye and clouding of the surface of the eye, usually going an opaque, blue-grey colour. Small blood vessels may be seen across the surface of the eye.

Causes Ulceration can be caused by damage to the cornea from scratches or foreign bodies in the eye, such as grass seeds, and infections of various kinds.

Owner action As with all eye conditions, early veterinary advice is essential. Bathing the eye with cotton wool dipped in warm water gently will help to soothe and ease the condition (see page 29).

Treatment Foreign bodies that may be the source of irritation should be flushed out of the eye. Antibiotic eye drops or cream will normally be used to counteract infection in the ulcerated area of the eye. Non-steroidal anti-inflammatory drugs may be given by mouth if the condition is particularly painful. Corticosteroidal treatment is not normally advised.

Related conditions Conjunctivitis (see page 29), periodic ophthalmia (see page 30), problems of the eyelid (see page 32), cataracts (see page 33) and tumours of the eye (see page 34).

 **DIAGNOSIS**

Ophthalmic examination of the eye is essential to differentiate this from other conditions that may have similar symptoms. Fluorescence staining, using a yellow dye that turns green when added to the eye, can be used to highlight any corneal ulceration. When the diagnosis with fluorescein is performed, the drainage of the tear ducts can also be checked.

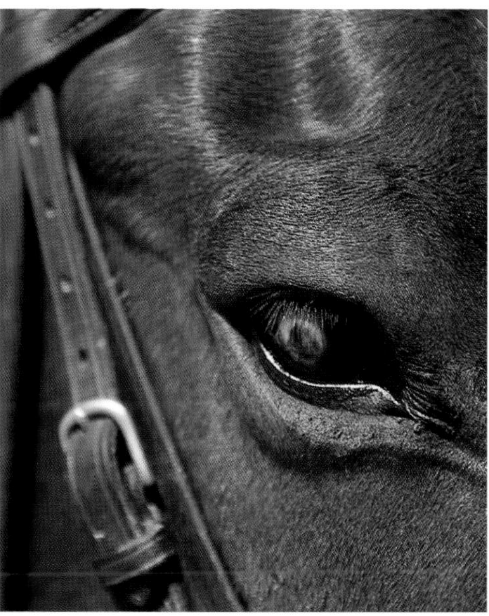

A corneal ulcer should be treated promptly before it causes any irreparable damage to the horse's eyesight.

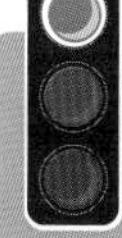

URGENCY INDICATOR

Urgent. Although this condition is not life threatening, there can be serious consequences for the eyesight and early treatment is necessary.

 **COST**

Quite low as long as complications are minimal.

Problems of the eyelid

The eyelid is the main protective mechanism for the eye. If the eyelid is damaged, or not functioning properly, damage may be caused to the eye itself.

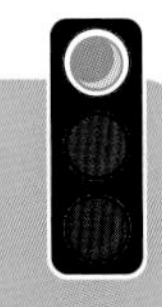

URGENCY INDICATOR

Urgent. All eye problems require immediate veterinary attention or advice to help prevent irreversible damage.

COST

Most conditions are fairly inexpensive to treat, unless they occur regularly. Often, though, they require a lot of time.

DIAGNOSIS

This may involve the use of a light source and magnifying lens, or perhaps an opthalmoscope to view into the eye. Soluble dye will identify if there is any damage to the cornea. A local anaesthetic may also be used to enable better examination of the eye.

ENTROPION

This is a condition where the margin of the eye turns in towards the eye. This will cause the eye lashes to scratch and irritate the eye.

Symptoms The condition causes excessive tear production and pain, and can be identified by careful inspection of the eye. In some cases there may be ulceration caused by the eyelashes scratching the surface of the cornea. It should not be mistaken for conjunctivitis (see page 29) or trauma.

Treatment Most cases can be resolved by simple treatment, turning the eyelid margins out and using antibiotic ointment. In more severe cases, injections into the eyelids to turn the eyelashes back out may be necessary. Occasionally surgical correction is required.

EYELID LACERATION

It is common for horses to cut their eyelids, whether on objects in the stable or outside.

Symptoms Sore, painful eye, with obvious cuts to the eyelid. May also be swelling.

Treatment If there is a good blood supply to the area and treatment is given early, healing is usually good. It is important to prevent the eyelids distorting during healing, because this may cause tear staining of the face and the complications that accompany this. With this type of injury it is important to assess the surface of the eye for any damage that may cause ulceration.

Always use fine materials in the care and repair of eyelids to reduce the chance of irritation during healing, so lessening the likelihood of the horse rubbing the wound and opening it again. Antibiotic ointment should be applied after repair to prevent any secondary infection and careful closing of the wound without removal of the skin of the eyelid is important.

WARNING Check looseboxes and paddocks for protruding sharp objects to prevent this type of injury occurring.

BLOCKED TEAR DUCTS

Tear ducts drain any lachrimation of the eye into the lachrymal duct, which comes out inside the end of the nostril. In cases of chronic eye inflammation or a foreign body in the eye, the tear duct may become blocked, which causes any lachrymal discharge to fall out of the eye and down the face, producing tear staining on the skin.

Symptoms Discharge from the eyes overflows down the face and causes tear staining.

Treatment Treatment is usually simple and involves flushing the tear ducts with an antibiotic and saline solution. Eyes that persistently discharge because of blocked tear ducts tend to attract flies, so secondary problems can arise.

Cataracts

Cataracts are opacities in the lens or its capsule, and can occur in just one or both eyes. They are more common in older horses, but foals may be born with congenital cataracts. Cataracts tend to cause a gradual loss of sight.

Symptoms Cataracts are difficult for an owner to observe unless they are extremely advanced, in which case a cloudy appearance to the lens will be visible if looked at carefully with a light.

Causes In the horse, cataracts are either congenital (the horse is born with them) or acquired as part of eye disease.

Owner action Any eye problems require urgent action in case there are less obvious underlying problems.

Treatment Cataracts in the adult horse are usually best left untreated, particularly if only one eye is affected and this does not obstruct vision to any great degree. If there is any doubt about the type of cataract, it is a good idea to monitor progress for safety reasons and arrange for your vet to re-examine the horse twice a year.

Related conditions Periodic ophthalmia (see page 30), uveitis and dislocation of the lens.

DIAGNOSIS

The horse may appear to have lost some of his normal vision. Examination with an ophthalmoscope will reveal the degree and extent of the cataract. It may also help to distinguish between congenital and acquired cataracts. Your vet will carry out an ophthalmological examination to confirm diagnosis and also to determine whether there are any additional underlying conditions.

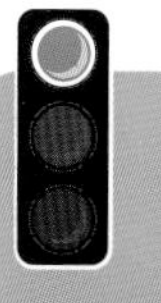

URGENCY INDICATOR

Urgent.

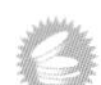

COST

If surgery is decided on it will be expensive, with only a guarded prognosis.

Tumours of the eye

Any structure in the eye has the potential to develop a tumour. Tumours are often visible as swellings, or can be a cause of loss of sight.

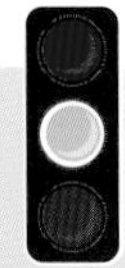

URGENCY INDICATOR

Non-urgent, but early diagnosis and treatment are recommended.

 **COST**

If surgery is required to remove either the tumour or the eye, it can be expensive.

Symptoms The eyeball may start to protrude or swellings and lumps may be noticed around the eyelids or on the third eyelid. These are all suggestive of eye tumour.

Causes The causes of many tumours are not known, but squamous cell carcinomas are likely to be affected by ultraviolet radiation.

 **DIAGNOSIS**

Clinical examination with an opthalmoscope and a biopsy of the lump may be required for diagnosis.

SARCOID TUMOURS

Sarcoid tumours of the eyelid are common in horses (see page 24). The treatment of sarcoid tumours in the eye varies, and can be complicated because of the different possible sites of the tumour and the sensitive nature of the tissue involved. Due to the recurrent nature of sarcoid tumours, eye sarcoids are potentially serious.

Treatment Local injections of BSG vaccine have been successful. In some cases, cryosurgery and surgical removal is useful, but the scarring effects of the treatment can affect eyelid function. Cytotoxic ointments have to be used extremely carefully and there is a danger that the preparation may be rubbed into the sensitive areas of the eye and cause damage.

SQUAMOUS CELL CARCINOMA

This tumour of the eyelid or third eyelid will often show as an ulcerative wound close to the margin of the eye or on the third eyelid, sometimes with swelling and discharge.

Treatment Treatment involves surgical excision, sometimes followed by radiation therapy. If the tumour affects the third eyelid, removal of the third eyelid is recommended.

IRIS MELANOMAS

Iris melanomas are uncommon and show up as an irregular mass on the margins of the pupil. These should be distinguished from iris cysts, which are round bodies attached to the iris and usually of little consequence.

Treatment The vet will usually recommend that no treatment be given.

PAPILLOMAS

Viral papillomas can sometimes be seen around the eyes of a young horse.

Treatment Usually no treatment is required and they tend to disappear with age. If papillomas persist, cryosurgery can be performed.

Problems of the outer ear

Infections in the ear are extremely rare. Occasionally, excessive wax production is seen, but cleaning of the ear should be undertaken only with great care and is usually totally unnecessary. Sometimes foreign bodies are found in the ear and the symptoms are head shaking and distress.

Symptoms Any swelling around the external ear, or abnormal aural discharge. Horses may become head shy, and will not allow their ears to be examined.

Causes As with most tumours, exact causes are not known.

DIAGNOSIS

Based on clinical examination. A biopsy may be required if a tumour is suspected.

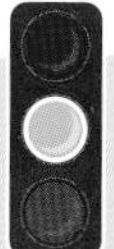

URGENCY INDICATOR

Fairly urgent, especially if there is a possible tumour or if the shape of the ear may be affected.

COST

Most ear problems requiring topical treatment will be fairly low cost. If surgery is required this will increase the costs.

EAR TUMOURS

The common tumours of the skin of the horse are found in the ear, the most common being sarcoids (see page 24). These can be a problem because of the irritation made by their mass. In addition, if the area of the sarcoid is between the bridle or head collar and the ear, problems can occur when tacking up and riding.

Treatment Treatment involves surgical excision, sometimes followed by radiation therapy.

AURAL PLAQUES

Aural plaques (papillary acanthosis) show up as a flat pink or pink-grey proliferative area on the inner side of the pinna. These are quite common and can extend into the ear canal itself, where wax and scale may accumulate. This condition rarely needs treatment and is unlikely to create a problem. In a few cases, secondary infection or inflammation occurs, and the waxy exudates associated with this condition also seem to attract biting flies. Owners often refer to this condition as fungal plaque, but there is no evidence that it is of fungal origin.

Treatment Treatment is inadvisable as it tends to cause head shyness.

SWEAT GLAND TUMOUR

This is an uncommon tumour of the sweat gland, which occurs mostly in older horses and is most commonly seen around the ear and the vulva as a single, firm, slow-growing nodule. It can be diagnosed by biopsy.

Treatment This involves surgical removal and the prognosis is good.

EAR INJURIES

The ear, like the eyelid, may often be torn when a horse rubs his head against a sharp object. This injury requires surgical repair to prevent unsightly scarring or curling of the ear surface.

Treatment Clean out any wounds with warm salty water, unless there is a possibility of the cleaning fluid going into the ear. Wounds may require stitching depending on their severity.

PROBLEMS OF THE MIDDLE AND INNER EAR

These are extremely rare, but occasionally occur due to trauma from fractures of the skull during falls or from septic meningitis. They cause symptoms such as head tilting, circling and falling over. Treatment of these cases depends upon the cause and is usually symptomatic.

Eating and drinking

Horses have evolved to live off a diet of grass and hay that is rich in cellulose. This has a symbiotic relationship with bacteria in the gut, the bacteria breaking down the cellulose into a form that horses are able digest. This process not only takes a long time but also requires a large fermentation chamber, called the caecum.

Grass is grasped by the incisors, causing the grass blades to break, and then ground by the cheek teeth into a digestible pulp. The tongue moves food from the incisors to the cheek teeth, and then to the back of the mouth. Food accumulates here just before it is swallowed. During this process, saliva from the salivary glands mixes with the food. Special enzymes in the saliva help with the breakdown of the food, which then passes down the oesophagus (a muscular tube) and is propelled into the stomach by a wave-like process, known as peristalsis. Food enters the stomach, where glands release more enzymes to aid digestion. Because their stomachs have one-way valves from the oesophagus, horses are unable to vomit.

The food then passes into the small intestine (another muscular tube containing a lining composed of glands) and moves through the tube, again by peristalsis. Enzymes produced by the liver and pancreas are released into the first part of the intestine through the glands, and these break down the food into three basic components: fats, proteins and carbohydrates.

These components are absorbed into the body, and transported in the blood and lymph to the liver. Here they are changed into different compounds that are used as energy. All the remaining food material now passes into the caecum, where the cellulose is fermented and broken down by micro-organisms into a digestible form. This material then passes into the large colon and small colon, which again are muscular tubes, and eventually passes into the rectum and anus, where it is excreted. During this process a lot of water is absorbed by the caecum and large colon.

Horses drink between 20 and 60 litres (5–13 gallons) a day, depending on the conditions, and they should have access to fresh water at all times.

For a diagram of the digestive system, see page 10.

Quick-reference guide to ailments in this chapter:

For **teeth and dental care**, see pages 38–39

For **eating problems**, see pages 40–42

For **problems which may be associated with eating**, see pages 43–45

For **worms and worming**, see pages 46–49

For **urinary and drinking problems**, see page 50

For **diarrhoea**, see page 51

Nutritional advice

The most important elements of a horse's diet are protein, vitamins and minerals. However, none of these can be used unless there is enough energy in the diet. Sources of energy are fibre, soluble carbohydrate (predominantly starch), fat and protein.

FIBRE

Fibre, the natural food of the horse, includes grass, hay, haylage, horsehage, alfalfa and oat-straw. It is made up of insoluble carbohydrate (cellulose, hemicellulose and lignin), sugars, starch and fats, which are found in the cell contents. Idle horses, barren mares and pregnant mares until the last third of pregnancy can be fed on fibre, as can horses in light to medium work. Fibre will also meet most of the energy requirements of all other classes of horse. Two factors limit how efficiently fibre can be used: the capacity of the digestive tract and the quality of the forage.

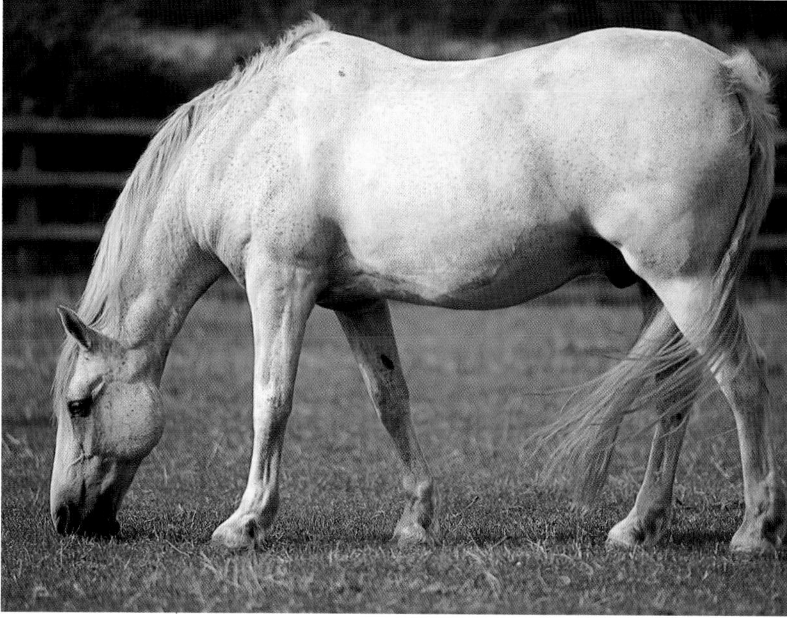

The amount of energy required by a horse will depend on his age and daily workload.

SOLUBLE CARBOHYDRATE (starch)

Soluble carbohydrates are found predominantly in grains (hard feed). Oats have the highest fibre content of grains, so they are safest. Maize is fed in many parts of the world, but it requires close monitoring because it has such a high energy content. Grains are an excellent source of energy because they are easily digested, but too much starch can kill the bacteria that live in the caecum and this leads to low-level diarrhoea, colic and, in extreme cases, laminitis. Starch needs to be fed in frequent, small amounts. Horses on this diet should always have access to fibre. It is especially important that grains are not fed on an empty stomach: make sure that the haynet is topped up before giving hard feed.

FAT

Unsaturated vegetable fats provide more energy per unit of weight than carbohydrates or proteins, and they are also digested very efficiently. They provide a short term boost of energy, and can be used as part of a food regime for competition horses.

PROTEIN

As the horse can only use protein for energy, it is not a preferred energy source and is often overfed. Forage supplies protein, often at levels that will satisfy even young, growing horses. Excess protein can cause sweating and raised heart and respiratory rates during endurance rides, and it is often associated with slower racing times in thoroughbreds. Increased drinking and excretion of ammonia, which is easily smelt, is often noticed. Increased urea and ammonia in the blood can cause digestive problems and nerve irritability in the horse.

VITAMINS AND MINERALS

These are found in good-quality hay and grass and in green leafy plants. Many commercial diets use a combination of the above. However short-blade fibre will be digested more quickly than long forage. Many commercial suppliers are now producing long-forage diets. When choosing a diet, it is better to get information from a nutritionist and from several food companies before deciding on their suitability.

Teeth and dental care

Horses' teeth have evolved over thousands of years to allow for effective grasping and chewing of the fibrous herbaceous food that makes up the vast majority of their natural diet. This causes relatively even wear on the horse's teeth, but with modern foodstuffs problems may arise.

Growth

Foals are born with two incisors and three cheek teeth. The rest of the teeth appear later, which means that a horse's age can be told by the state of his teeth. The upper and lower jaws have the same number of teeth. An adult horse has six incisors, two canines or tushes (these are normally absent in the mare), 12 cheek teeth and sometimes one or two wolf teeth.

Horses' teeth are hyposodont (long-crowned), which means that they are extruded (pushed out) constantly through adult life by 2–3mm (⅛in) a year. The teeth do not grow continuously as in some other species (rodents, for example), but on average most teeth have a reserve of 7–10cm (3–4in). When a tooth reaches the limit of the reserve, it falls out.

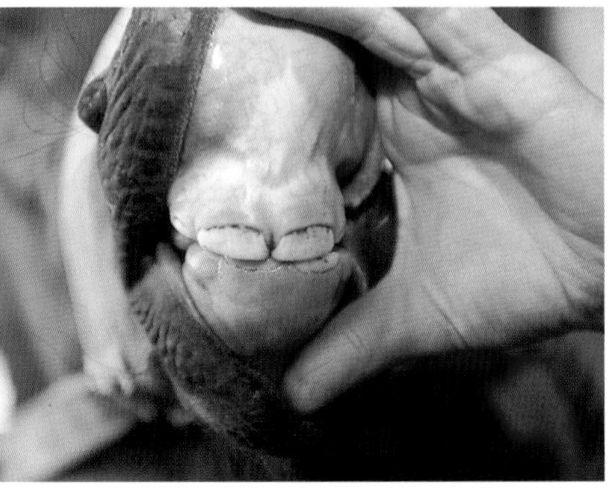

Foal teeth: two central incisors are there, with the two incisors behind them just coming through.

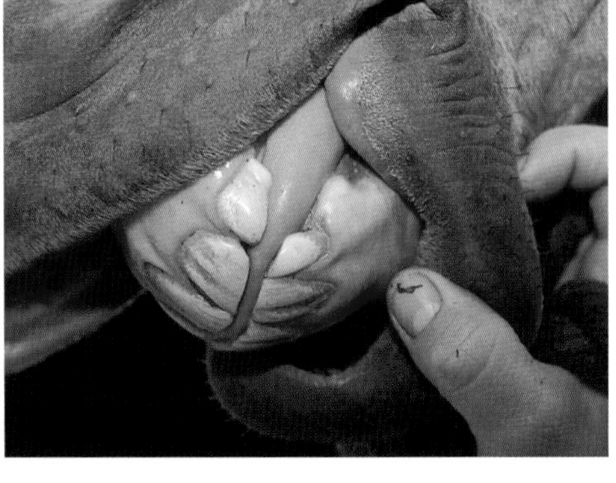

A 5-year-old's teeth, with the corner incisor just coming into wear.

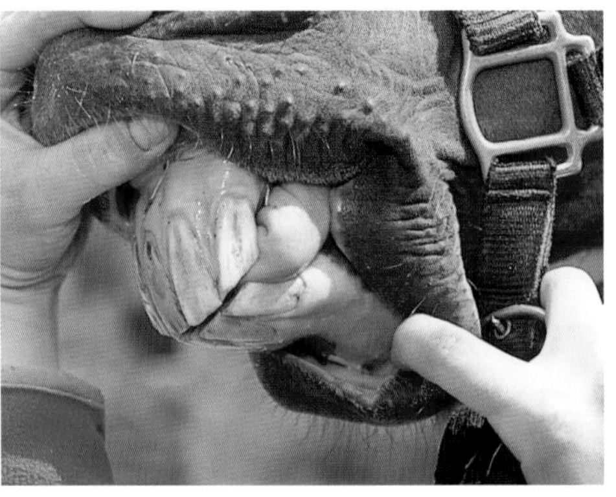

A 15-year-old's teeth: at this age the angle at which the horse's teeth meet is much greater.

Tooth formation

The right and left mandibular teeth (lower jaw) are closer together than the right and left maxillary teeth (upper jaw). This means that the maxillary teeth overlap the mandibular teeth on their outside surface, and the mandibular teeth overlap the maxillary teeth on their inside surface. Some horses' maxillary teeth overlap the mandibular at the front, and the mandibular teeth overlap the maxillary teeth at the back. This can lead to the formation of hooks on the front maxillary teeth and the back mandibular teeth.

In the wild, the constant grinding of the teeth on different types of fibrous herbaceous food material would have caused fairly even wear. Unfortunately, this no longer happens as efficiently with modern foodstuffs and the following problems can occur:

- uneven wear of the tops of the teeth
- formation of hooks on the outer surface of the maxillary teeth and the inner surface of the mandibular teeth.

Wolf teeth

Wolf teeth occur in the bit-seat area. If they are on the outside of the gum, are very big or move they cause discomfort when the cheek or bit is pushed into them. This is especially obvious when a horse bends his head forward, causing the maxillary teeth to move in front of the mandibular teeth and increasing the pressure on them. Not all wolf teeth cause problems.

A wolf tooth is normally removed under sedation and local anaesthetic is injected around the tooth. It takes at least two weeks for the wound to heal, and the horse should not be ridden during this time.

Routine rasping

Teeth should be routinely examined every six months or at least once a year. The horse's tongue can be held and pressed into the roof of the mouth and to the side to allow the teeth and gums to be seen with a torch. A gag may be used to allow all the teeth to be felt, which makes a more thorough examination possible. If any teeth have hooks or are sharp, the teeth should be rasped.

Usually, the outer surface of the maxillary teeth and the inner surface of the mandibular teeth, and the front maxillary teeth and the back mandibular teeth, are rasped to remove hooks. A variety of different rasps is used – thin and thick, long and short – and electric burs may also be used.

During rasping the horse should be held over the bridge of the nose to prevent him lifting his head. If the horse is scared of rasping or a lot of work is necessary, it may be better for him to be sedated to allow a more thorough job and for the safety of the horse and handlers. Only a vet or a qualified horse dentist should carry out rasping.

Bit seating

A bit pushes the cheek upwards and inwards. It is, therefore, important that any contact points are smooth. Often the maxillary teeth are rounded to allow better seating of the bit.

THE TEETH

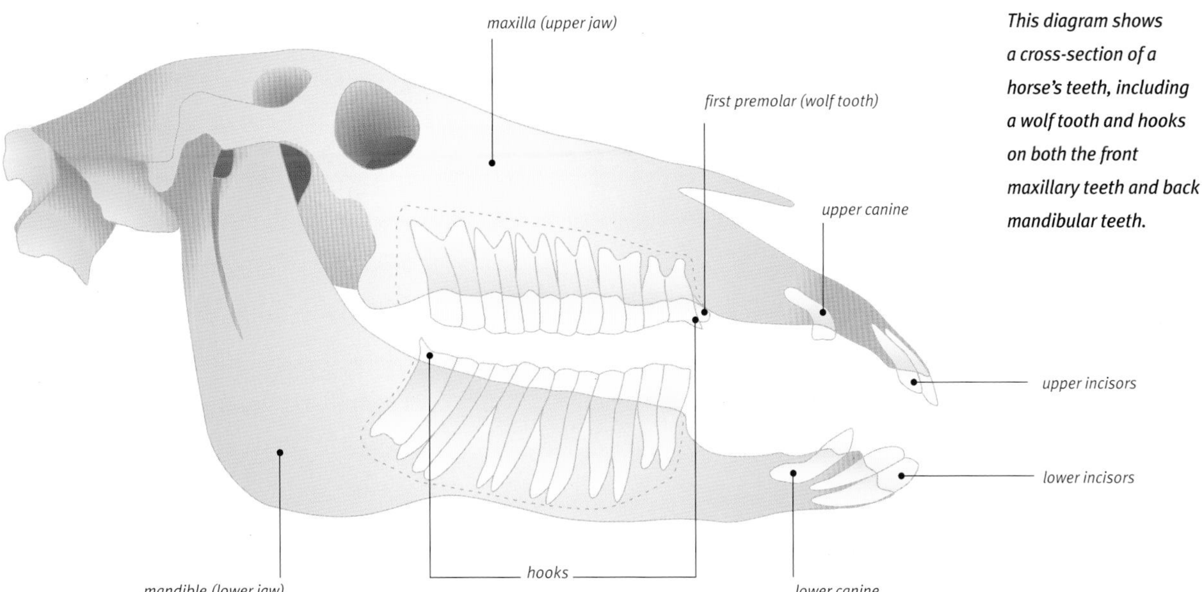

This diagram shows a cross-section of a horse's teeth, including a wolf tooth and hooks on both the front maxillary teeth and back mandibular teeth.

Teeth problems

Regular attention to your horse's teeth is very important in order to maintain good health and spot any potential problems at an early stage.

DEVELOPMENTAL DEFECTS

Parrot mouth The upper jaw overshoots the lower jaw. In thoroughbreds it is said to occur only if there is no apposition of the incisors. In other breeds it is diagnosed if there is malocclusion of the incisors.

Polydontia This occurs where there are more teeth than there should be, often an extra cheek tooth. If the extra teeth are causing a problem, they should be removed. Otherwise they should be monitored closely.

Retained deciduous incisors Sometimes these can cause the permanent incisors to be displaced. They are easily removed.

DENTAL ERUPTION CYSTS

The second and third cheek teeth are squashed during their eruption, and this causes a reaction in the surrounding bone. This can be felt under the mandible as firm swellings. As the horse continues to grow, the jaw elongates, which normally causes the swellings to disappear spontaneously. If the swellings do not disappear or start to discharge, a vet should examine the horse.

Parrot mouth can cause eating difficulties if the horse is not given regular dental attention.

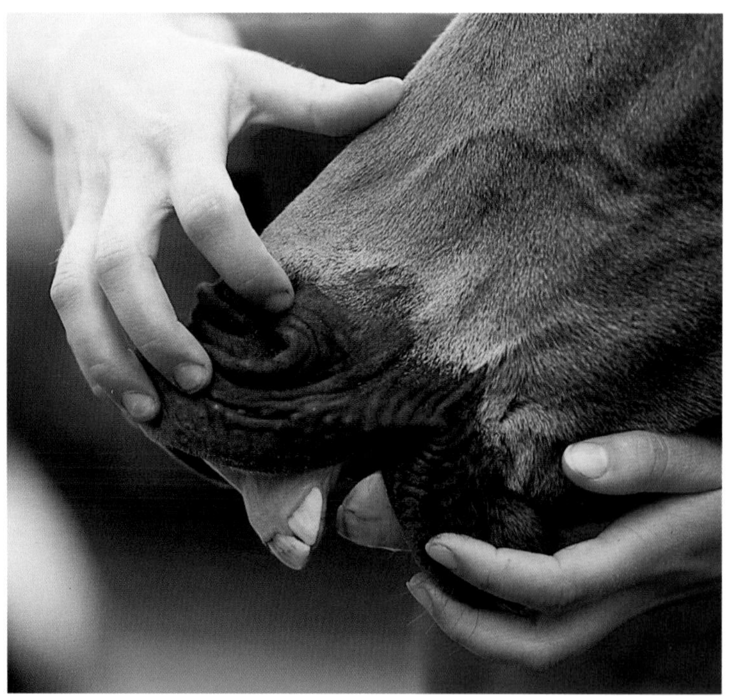

 **DIAGNOSIS**

An examination of the mouth will be needed. A gag is usually used to keep the mouth open. X-rays may be taken to assess the extent of damage to the root of the tooth or infection. If there is not an obvious problem, blood tests may be taken to determine if any other body systems are involved.

SHEARMOUTH

Hooks develop on the outer surface of the maxillary teeth, the inner surface of the mandibular teeth and on the front maxillary teeth and back mandibular teeth. If they are not routinely rasped flat, the teeth are unable to move from left to right in a grinding motion. This causes the formation of a slope on the top of the teeth, and in time this allows the jaw to move only in a scissor-like shearing action.

WAVEMOUTH

This is caused by uneven rates of wear and eruption over all the teeth. This is often seen in the presence of shearmouth and periodontal disease, and if a tooth is lost. It is common in older animals.

ABRASION

This occurs when the teeth are subjected to unnatural constant wear, such as crib biting.

DENTAL CALCULUS

This is not as significant in horses as it is in humans. Horses often get calculus on the tushes and other teeth, and it should be removed by the vet.

Eating problems

Eating problems are a common disorder in the horse, especially in older ones. They have the potential to be very serious unless diagnosed early as they can cause problematic weight loss.

Symptoms Reluctance to eat, eating slowly, dropping food from mouth when eating (quidding), smelly breath (halitosis), playing in the water bucket when eating, selectively feeding on easily chewed food and losing weight.

Causes Developmental defects and eruption cysts (see page 40), hooks and tooth infections (see below).

Owner action If any of the symptoms are seen the horse should be examined by a vet.

Treatment Treatment depends on the cause, but usually includes tooth rasping. If there is an infected tooth, a course of antibiotics may be needed and possibly removal of the tooth. Fractured teeth are normally removed. Tooth removal normally requires a general anaesthetic, unless it is an old wobbly tooth that may be easily pulled out. Afterwards, the horse's feed may need to be changed to a foodstuff that he can chew more easily.

DIAGNOSIS

An examination of the mouth will be needed. A gag is usually used to keep the mouth open. X-rays may be taken to assess the extent of any damage. If there is not an obvious problem, blood tests may be taken to determine if any other body systems are involved.

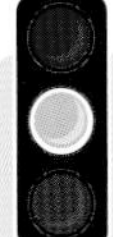

URGENCY INDICATOR

Fairly urgent, especially if the horse is losing weight.

COST

Routine dentistry is relatively cheap, but the more work that is needed the higher the cost.

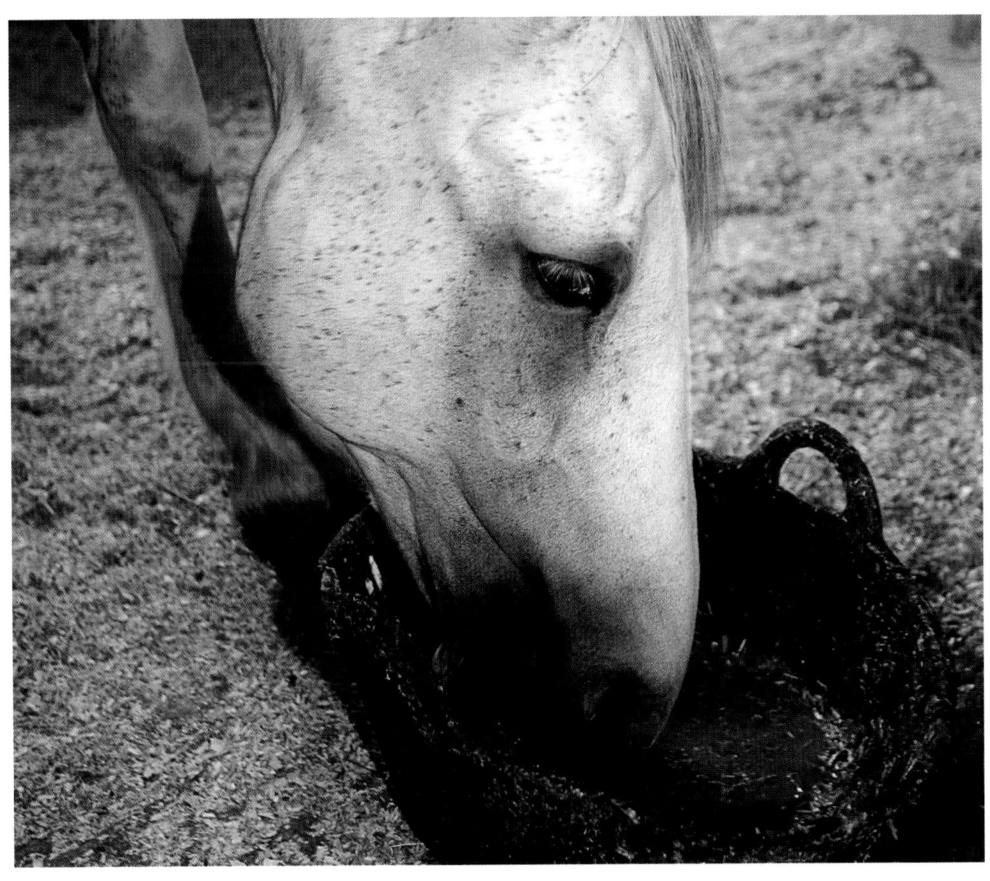

Monitor your horse's eating habits, as any changes may indicate an underlying problem that requires attention.

The thin horse

The ribs and vertebrae should not be visible in the normal horse (although ribs may be visible in some fit race horses). Young and old horses have the ability to lose condition very rapidly, and should be watched closely.

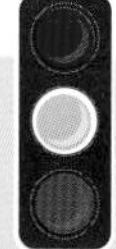

URGENCY INDICATOR

Fairly urgent to prevent further weight loss.

COST

This will depend on how obvious the cause is, and how many tests will be required.

Symptoms Visible ribs and possibly visible vertebrae. This may be accompanied by diarrhoea, quidding, constipation, yellowing of the mucus membranes (jaundice), swelling in the legs and under the belly (oedema), colic symptoms or worms.

Causes Problems eating, poor-quality food, liver problems, digestion problems, tumours, worms, pain, grass sickness, stomach ulcers.

Owner action Try to determine whether the horse is thin because he is not eating properly due to, for example, teeth problems, competition from other horses for food or not enough food. Make sure worming is up to date.

Determine whether the horse has diarrhoea or is constipated. Work out a time scale over which the horse has lost weight. When feeding hard feed, make sure that the haynet has been filled first, so that there is fibre in the gut before the hard feed is offered.

Treatment Depends on the cause.

DIAGNOSIS

The horse may need a full clinical examination. Blood tests and faecal samples may be taken.

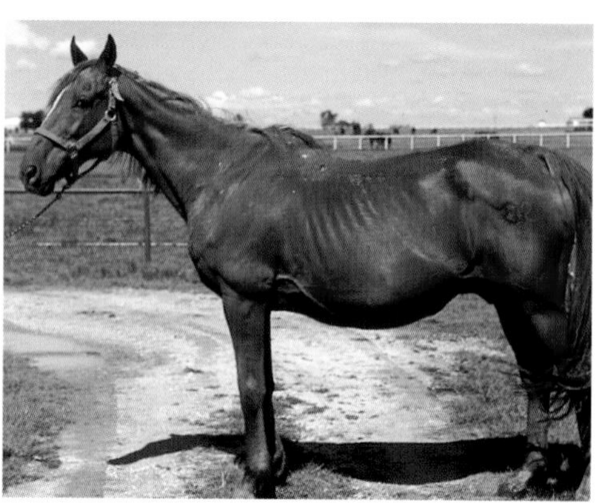

Visible ribs and poor condition are the most obvious indicators of a thin horse.

The fat horse

A horse in good condition should have palpable ribs, although not visible, and a difference in definition between the thorax and the back of the abdomen. Overweight horses are becoming increasingly common.

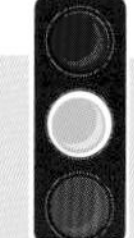

URGENCY INDICATOR

Fairly urgent to prevent further weight gain and laminitis or associated problems.

COST

Depends on the tests needed and any other complicating problems.

DIAGNOSIS

Based on full clinical examination. Blood tests may be used to assess blood sugar levels.

Symptoms No palpable ribs or waist.

Causes Usually overfeeding, although it can be caused by sugar metabolism problems.

Owner action Gradually cut out any concentrates, feed lower-quality forage and increase exercise. Be careful to watch for laminitis, to which overweight ponies are very prone.

Treatment Specific treatment is needed only if a cause has been identified, otherwise a gradual cut-down on food is all that will be required.

Choke

This is a common problem often associated with feeding, when impacted food or foreign material becomes blocked in the oesophagus. The symptoms are often very distressing and alarming.

Symptoms Severe distress, extension of the head and neck, saliva and food material pouring from the nose, reluctance to eat or drink.

Causes Often follows feeding, if the food is eaten too quickly or not chewed correctly (see page 41). The oesophagus can become obstructed by large particles of food, such as big pieces of carrot or pelleted feed. There may be problems with the mobility of the oesophagus, particularly if the horse is fed too soon after sedation.

Owner action Remove food but leave water. Massage the left side of the neck, in sweeping movements from under the chin to the base of the neck. Phone immediately for veterinary advice and assistance.

Treatment Depending on the severity of the condition, a vet may give an antispasmodic injection, which relaxes the smooth muscle in the oesophagus and allows the obstruction to pass. A stomach tube may be passed to lavage (wash out) the blockage with water. Sedation may be given to keep the head lowered and prevent the horse from breathing in saliva and food. Antibiotics may be given to help prevent secondary respiratory infections resulting from the inhalation of food and saliva. Analgesics may be given to reduce pain. Sometimes it may take repeated veterinary visits to dislodge the obstruction. After the obstruction has been cleared, the oesophagus may be viewed through an endoscope to check for any problems or damage to the oesophagus.

DIAGNOSIS

Based on clinical signs, and the inability to pass a stomach tube. Most horses will have to be sedated to allow a stomach tube to be passed.

Related conditions Strangles (see page 55), colic (see pages 44–45), cleft palate in foals, guttural pouch disorders (see page 59), tumours and pharyngeal problems.

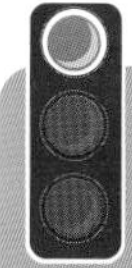

URGENCY INDICATOR

Urgent: a horse cannot eat or drink until a choke has cleared.

COST

Fairly expensive, as often needs repeat visits. Very expensive if an oesophageal tear occurs.

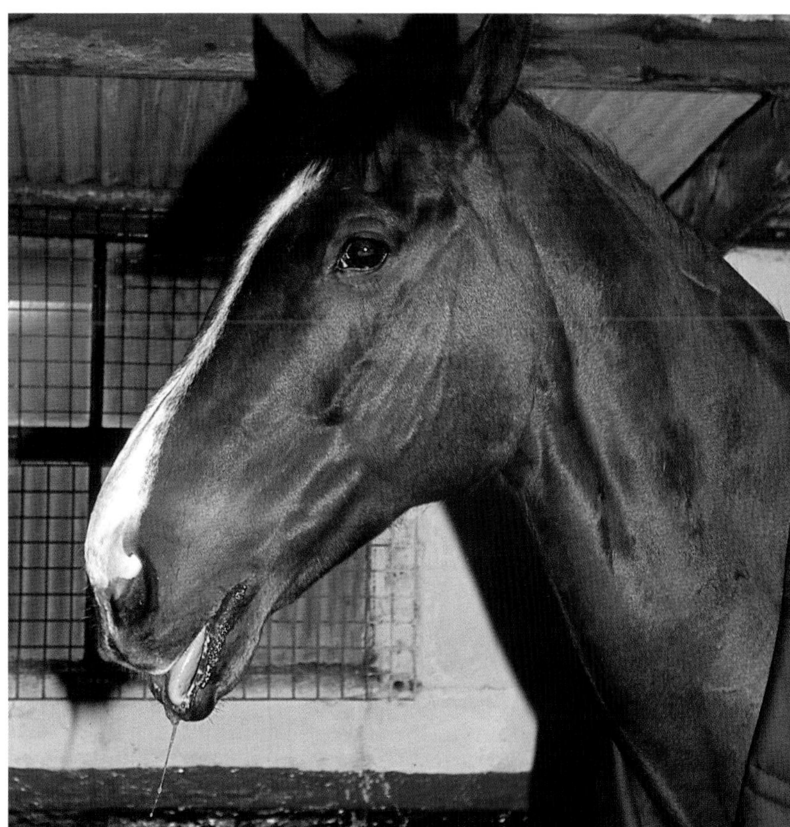

A choking horse can become very distressed and cough up mucus.

Colic

Any form of abdominal pain results in colic, although there are numerous possible causes. It is is a serious condition and should be treated straight away.

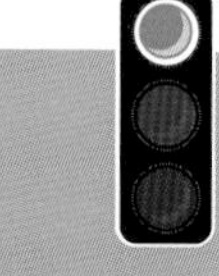

URGENCY INDICATOR

Very urgent – a horse with severe colic requiring surgery should be operated on as soon as possible.

COST

This can vary depending on the type of colic – mild colic that resolves itself will cost very little, but surgery can be very expensive.

Symptoms Belly watching, pawing the ground, pacing, rolling, lying down, kicking at the belly, food regurgitation from the nostrils, flared nostrils, increased respiratory rate, pale/blue gums, excessive urge to urinate, refusal of food and water, sweating.

Causes Most causes of colic are not known, but box rest, excitability, change in food or the weather and recent worming may all cause problems. Infection and worms have also been implicated in colic.

Owner action Phone your vet immediately. Remove all food from the stable, and if possible put down non-edible bedding. Make sure the bedding is deep so that the horse will not hurt himself by rolling. Walking may help to settle the horse, but if he is trying to roll he is best left in the stable, where he cannot harm himself or the handler. Allowing a horse to roll will not cause him to twist his stomach: a horse with a twisted stomach will roll because of the pain that he is in! Try to make a note of any changes in husbandry, such as worming dates or a change of food or fields.

DIAGNOSIS

The vet will perform a full clinical examination, paying a lot of attention to gum colour, heart and respiratory rate, and gut sounds. A rectal examination will often be performed, which enables abnormal structures to be felt. A stomach tube may be passed to determine if there is excess fluid or gas in the stomach, which would suggest that there might be an obstruction.

Treatment This depends on the cause. Antispasmodic injections can calm muscle spasm and cramping, analgesia will bring pain relief, stomach tubing with liquid paraffin may help move a blockage, intravenous fluid therapy may relieve blockages, and probiotics, which restore gut flora. In serious cases, surgical correction of twisted intestines may be necessary.

Related conditions Choke (see page 43), setfast (see page 78), twisted testicles, inflammation of any of the abdominal organs, urinary problems (see page 50), post-foaling complications (see page 106), peritonitis and laminitis (see page 74).

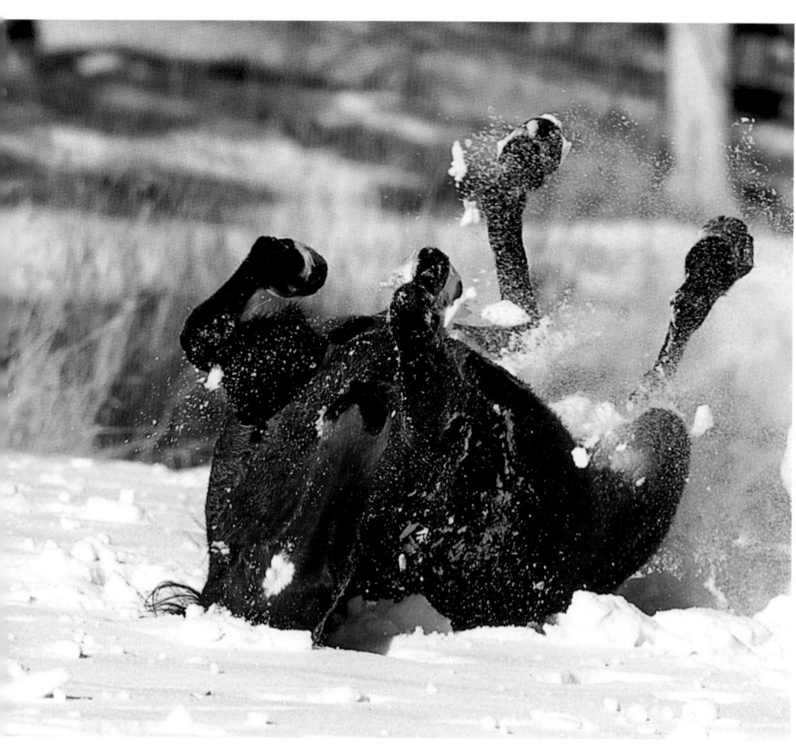

Colic is often evident as winter arrives and there is a change in the horse's usual diet.

Forms of colic

The main forms of colic are discussed below. There are also some miscellaneous causes, including wind sucking, sand colic, worms (excessive tapeworm burdens cause blockages) and migrating worm larvae.

SPASMODIC COLIC

This is a form of indigestion and has many causes. It is common in animals about to compete or hunt if they are excited. Different foods, worming or changes in the environment can also cause it.

Treatment Usually responds quickly to anti-spasmodics and mild analgesics

IMPACTED COLIC

If there is a severe change in the motility of the intestines, food in the large colon can stop moving and then cause a blockage. A common place for this is the pelvic flexure, which is a narrow area of the large colon. Impactions (blockages of rough, fibrous material) may also be a symptom of grass sickness (see below). These are common in box-rested horses.

Treatment Analgesics, water and liquid paraffin can be given by stomach tube, and intravenous fluids by injection. If the impaction does not respond to treatment, surgery may be necessary.

TWISTED INTESTINES

This is a very severe form of colic and happens very quickly. Unfortunately, due to the design of the small intestine, it easily twists around itself or gets caught in other parts of the abdomen. Older horses often have fatty lumps on stalks, which the intestine can also twist around.

Treatment The only corrective treatment is surgery, without which the horse will die, and if surgery is not an option the horse should be euthanased as soon as possible on humane grounds. As soon as the intestine twists, the blood supply to the twist is cut off. With no blood, the twist receives no oxygen, so starts to die. As this happens, toxins within the twisted intestine leak into the abdomen. The other main problem with a twist is that the horse continues to salivate, so the stomach continues to fill with fluid. Because there is a twist, the fluid builds up in the stomach, and because the horse cannot be sick, the stomach bursts. Obviously, both these problems lead to a very painful death.

GRASS SICKNESS

This affects horses and ponies at grass. The cause is still not properly understood, and not all the animals in a field will be affected. It causes varying symptoms. An acute form will involve twisted intestines, often accompanied by patchy sweating and trembling of the skin. The other chronic form causes severe weight loss, often accompanied by impactions.

Treatment Neither form is treatable and will result in death.

Worms

There are four major types of internal parasite: the large redworm, small redworm, tapeworm and bots. All of these live in the digestive tract of the horse.

LARGE REDWORM

(Large strongyles; *Strongylus vulgaris, S. edentatus, S. equinis, Triodontophorus* spp.)

Eggs pass out in the dung. These hatch into larvae, which survive on the pasture and are then eaten by the horse. Once digested, they travel through blood vessels or the liver, before becoming adults in the large intestine and producing eggs. They can damage blood vessels in the abdomen as well as cause inflammation of the lining of the intestine. All wormers will kill this worm.

SMALL REDWORM

(Small strongyles; *Cyathastome* spp.)

The life cycle is the same as that of the large redworm. Once ingested, larvae burrow into the wall of the large intestine, where they undergo several larval stages, then emerge to become adults. Large numbers picked up in late summer and autumn can become dormant (encysted) in the gut wall. They can all emerge simultaneously in late winter or early spring, causing enormous damage, which leads to severe diarrhoea, weight loss and sometimes death, especially in foals and yearlings. A five-day course of benzimidazole or moxidectin will kill this worm and its larval stages.

TAPEWORM

(*Anoplocephala perfoliata*)

Eggs in the dung are eaten by a forage mite, which lives in pasture, bedding and hay. While grazing, the horse eats the mite containing the larval stage of the tapeworm, which becomes an adult in the lower part of the small intestine and ileocaecal junction where, in large numbers, they may cause inflammation and colic. Pyrantel and praziquantel will kill this worm.

BOTS

(*Gasterophillus* spp.)

Bots are the larval stage of the bot fly, which lays creamy-yellow eggs on the legs and body of the horse in summer and early autumn. These are licked off, the larvae hatch out and are swallowed. They remain attached to the stomach lining over the winter, where they can cause irritation and inflammation. Ivermectin will kill these worms.

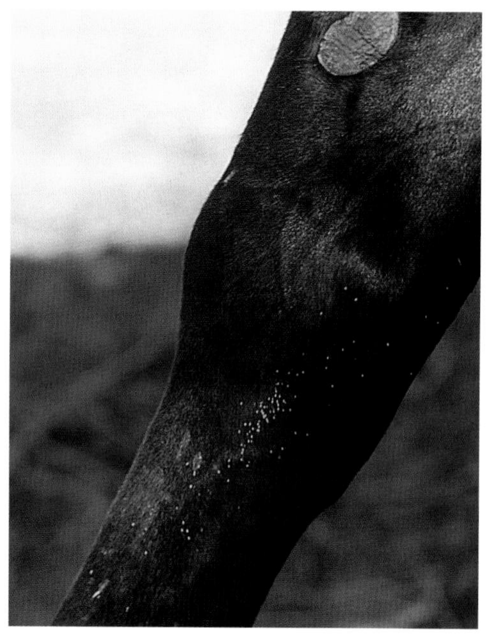

Bot eggs are laid on the horse's legs and body by the bot fly in the summer and early autumn.

MINOR TYPES

Lungworm (*Dictyocaulus arnfieldi*) The lungworm is a parasite of donkeys, in which there may be no clinical signs, but eggs are passed out in the donkey's faeces. Horses grazing in fields where donkeys have grazed can pick up the larvae. The parasite can cause coughing and respiratory problems, though only rarely do the worms become adult and produce eggs in the horse. Ivermectin is the only effective treatment for lungworm.

Pinworm *(Oxyuris equi)* The female worm lives in the large intestine. When it is ready to breed it crawls out through the rectum to the anus, where it lays clusters of eggs on the skin around the anus and under the tail. The eggs are irritating; horses become itchy and rub their tails. All worming drugs will deal effectively with this worm.

Roundworm *(Parascaris equorum)* These large worms are mainly a problem of foals and are found in the small intestine. They cause loss of appetite, unthriftiness and a potbelly. If there are enough worms they can cause colic or may actually cause blockages in the intestine. The worms infect foals from one year to a next, so cleanliness is the most important factor in prevention. All wormers will kill this worm.

Threadworm *(Strongyloides westeri)* This is a small, fine worm found in the intestines of foals. The foal is infected from the mother's milk. The parasites can cause a range of symptoms, ranging from lethargy, loss of condition and retained winter coat, loss of performance and diarrhoea to colic and even occasionally death. Benzimidazole and ivermectin are effective at killing the worm.

WORM CONTROL

Effective worm control combines pasture management with strategic use of the different types of wormers available. Not all wormers control the same parasites and some parasites are more effectively killed at certain times of the year. The cycle of re-infection of the horse from the pasture and contamination of the pasture from the horse has to be broken. The worming programme is based on the strategic use of specific wormers, plus routine worming, through the grazing season from mid-spring to early autumn. It is recommended that only one type of routine wormer is used each year as this helps to prevent the build-up of resistance in the worm population.

An effective worming programme needs to be combined with sound management of the pasture.

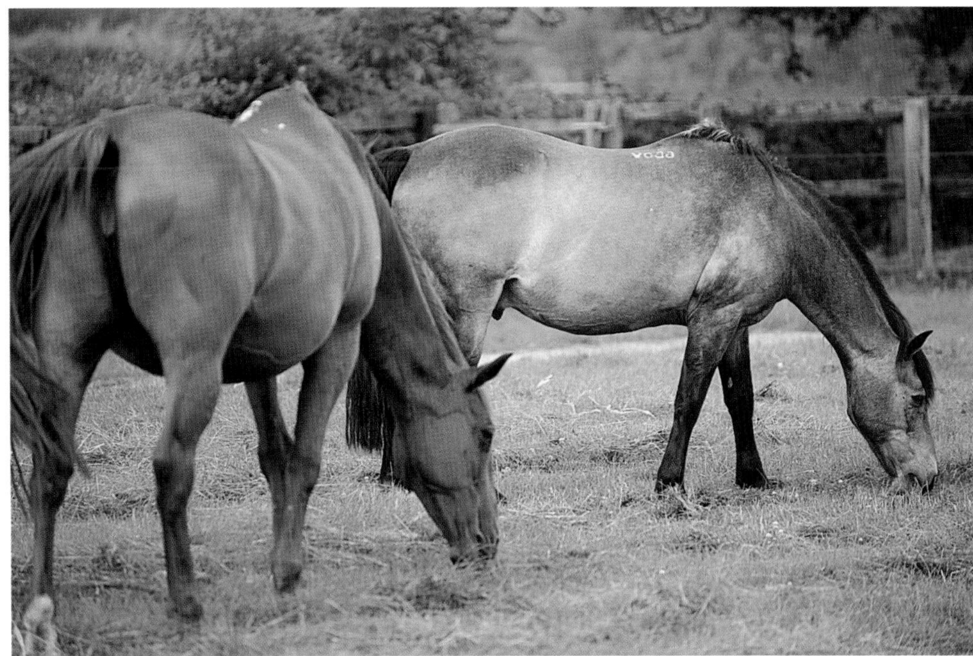

The risk of faecal contamination of pastures is increased by having large numbers of horses on small pastures.

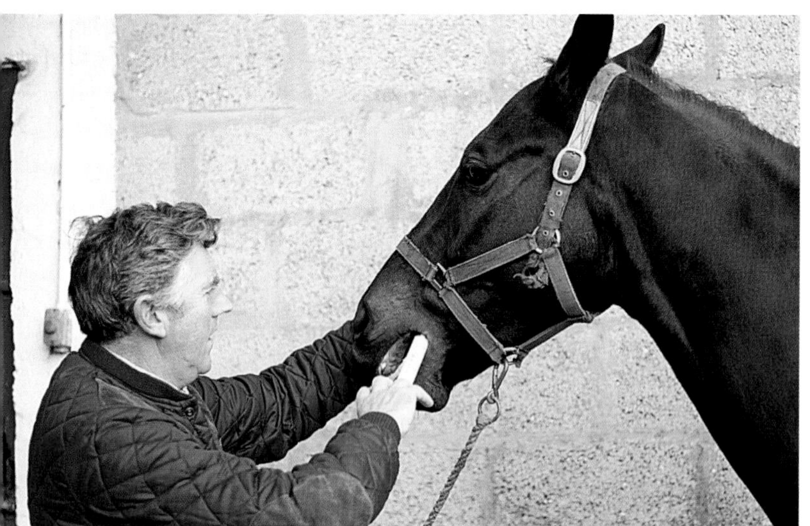

Most wormers are given in paste or gel form, syringed directly into the horse's mouth. Some are available in powder or liquid form to be added to the feed.

Pasture contamination

Dosing with wormer in early or mid-spring will reduce pasture contamination at the start of the grazing season.

Pasture management

Removing dung from the paddocks twice a week in summer and once a week from early winter to mid-spring has been shown to reduce the worm population considerably and will also increase the areas of grass for grazing.

If possible, move your horse to a new and ideally clean pasture 12–24 hours after worming. Mixed grazing with cattle or sheep reduces the number of worm larvae on the grass and also improves the quality of the pasture. Harrowing in dry weather causes larvae to die.

Clean grazing for mares with foals is advised – clean for small redworms is five months and for roundworms 12 months with no horses on. Fields that have been grown and cut for silage or hay are ideal first pastures for foals.

Dose

Always make sure you give the correct dose. It is easy to underestimate your horse's weight.

New horses

It is safest to assume that new horses are carrying worms. Ideally, treat them straight away with a wormer for encysted small redworm and a week later for tapeworm. Stabling for the first 48 hours and burning or composting the faeces will reduce the risk of contaminating the pastures.

Stable yards

Livery stables, riding schools and yards are advised to have a worming regime, with all horses being treated on the same day.

WORMERS

Five groups of wormers are commonly used:

1. Pyrantel

A single dose is effective against adult large and small redworms, pinworms and roundworms but not larval stages.

The dosing interval is four to six weeks, after which another wormer should be used.

A double dose is the only effective treatment for tapeworms and should be done most effectively in early spring and early autumn at the end of housing and grazing seasons.

2. Benzimadazole

At normal dose rates this will control adult and immature stages, but not migrating or dormant stages, of large and small redworms.

The dosing interval is six to eight weeks.

A five-day course of benzimadazole controls the inhibited stages of small redworms in the wall of the hind gut, which can cause so much damage when they emerge *en masse*. The recommended time to give this course is autumn, then once again in early spring.

3. Ivermectin

At normal dose rates this is effective against adult and immature large and small redworms (but not inhibited small redworms), lungworms, pinworms, roundworms and *S. westeri*, and is also the only effective treatment for bots, which are most effectively treated in early winter.

The dosing interval is eight to ten weeks.

4. Moxidectin

This should eliminate 80 per cent of developing encysted small redworms but not the dormant stages of small redworms. It is also effective in the treatment and control of large redworms (both adult and arterial stages), roundworms, pinworms and bots.

The dosing interval is 13 weeks.

It prevents re-infection with small redworms for two weeks after dosing and is also useful for suppressing egg production in the faeces for 90 days after dosing, which helps reduce pasture contamination. Used in late autumn or early winter, it will be well-timed to eliminate bots. In early to mid-spring it will reduce the contamination of the pasture by eggs in the faeces. It can be used in foals over four months of age and in pregnant mares.

5. Praziquantel

This is not available on its own but is combined with ivermectin. This makes an effective tapeworm treatment, as well as being effective against large redworms and bots. It is used seasonally.

WORM CONTROL PROGRAMME CALENDAR

Month	Worm problem	Wormer product	Preventative measures
Midwinter			
Late winter	*Encysted redworm larvae*	*5-day benzimidazole course or moxidectin*	*To reduce pasture contamination at turnout*
Early spring	*Tapeworm*	*Pyrantel or praziquantel*	
Mid-spring		*Any*	*Routine worming*
Late spring		*Any*	*Routine worming*
Early summer		*Any*	*Routine worming*
Midsummer		*Any*	*Routine worming*
Late summer		*Any*	*Routine worming*
Early autumn	*Tapeworm*	*Pyrantel or praziquantel*	
Mid-autumn	*Encysted redworm larvae*	*5-day benzimidazole course or moxidectin*	
Late autumn			
Early winter	*Bots*	*Ivermectin*	

Urinary problems

Horses do not commonly suffer from urinary problems, and unfortunately many are probably missed simply because when horses are at grass it is difficult to see if they have a problem.

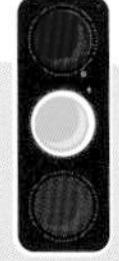

URGENCY INDICATOR

Fairly urgent.

COST

Initial urine tests are fairly inexpensive, but if further tests such as endoscopy are required then costs will begin to mount up.

Symptoms Pain on urination, straining to urinate, discoloured urine, smelly urine, increased or decreased urination.

Causes Cystitis, bladder tumours, urinary stones, kidney infections, ruptured bladder (newborn foals).

Owner action Try to collect a urine sample. Normal urine varies in colour from light yellow to orange and is often cloudy. Make sure your horse has access to plenty of water.

Treatment Treatment depends on the cause. The horse may be given antibiotics, and the vet may recommend a change of feed. If urinary stones are present, adding feed supplements may dissolve them or they may need to be removed surgically.

Related conditions Colic (see pages 44–45) and setfast (see page 78).

DIAGNOSIS

The horse will need a full clinical examination by the vet. Urine and blood samples may be taken. Rectal palpation and endoscopy of the urethra or the bladder may be carried out.

Drinking-related problems

Individual horses will drink different amounts of water, but a normal horse will drink between two and four buckets of water a day – any more or less may suggest problems.

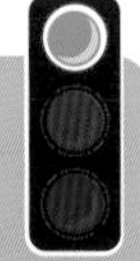

URGENCY INDICATOR

Urgent, because of the importance of underlying conditions and the possibility of dehydration.

COST

Depends on what tests are needed.

Symptoms Any change in normal water consumption. This may be accompanied by increased or decreased urination, colicky symptoms, a long curly coat or loss of appetite.

Causes The most common cause is reduced drinking because of poor water quality or taste – for example, high chlorine – or lack of available water. Other less common causes are Cushing's disease, diabetes, colic, pyschogenic polydipsia and renal failure.

Owner action Make sure that your horse has a good supply of fresh water and always monitor the amount drunk each day, especially in hot weather and when your horse is competing.

Treatment Treatment depends on the cause.

DIAGNOSIS

A veterinary examination may be necessary, and the vet will want to know the history of the horse. Blood and urine samples may be taken.

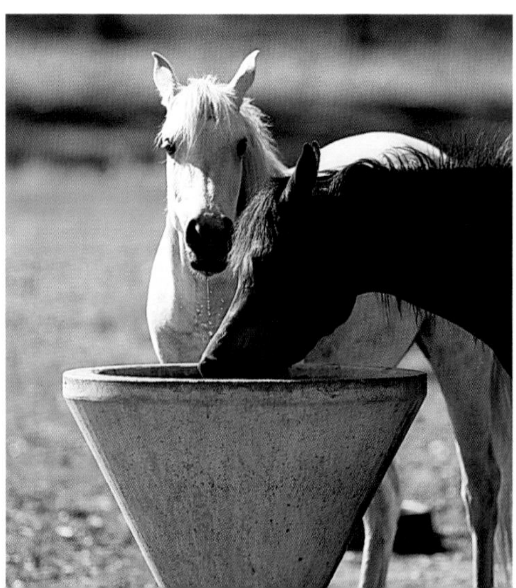

Note any changes in your horse's normal drinking pattern.

Diarrhoea

Diarrhoea is caused by a rapid movement of food through the gastro-intestinal tract, which prevents the normal absorption of water, nutritive elements and electrolytes, and produces very watery faeces, often of an increased frequency.

Symptoms Loose or watery faeces, which are often accompanied by faecal staining of the hind legs and tail. Colicky symptoms may also be present.

Causes Overfeeding of carbohydrates, infections such as salmonella, worms, increased gut motility, such as is caused by spasmodic colic, antibiotic use, acorn ingestion, tumours, liver problems or stomach ulcers.

Owner action Quarantine the horse to prevent the problem spreading to other horses. Wash your hands and clothes regularly to stop possible zoonotic spread of infectious agents, such as salmonella. Make sure horses are wormed regularly and correctly. Gradually stop providing any concentrates and feed good-quality fibre.

Treatment This depends on the cause, but may include antibiotics, probiotics and worming. Also, drugs to coat and protect the stomach and to stop the production of stomach enzymes may be used.

Related conditions Spasmodic colic (see pages 44–45), infections, stomach ulcers, worms and worming (see pages 46–49).

DIAGNOSIS

A full clinical examination is made. Faecal (dung) samples may be taken for analysis and worm and larvae counts. Blood samples may be taken to check liver function and to determine if there is damage to the digestive system. Rectal biopsies and glucose absorption tests may be taken to determine if the problem is related to the large or small intestine. Endoscopy may be used to view the lining of the stomach. Samples of the fluid in the abdomen may be taken.

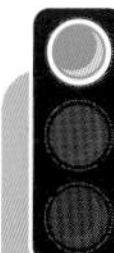

URGENCY INDICATOR

Urgent. Diarrhoea is very serious and can lead to rapid dehydration.

COST

Depends on the cause. The more tests required, the higher the cost will be.

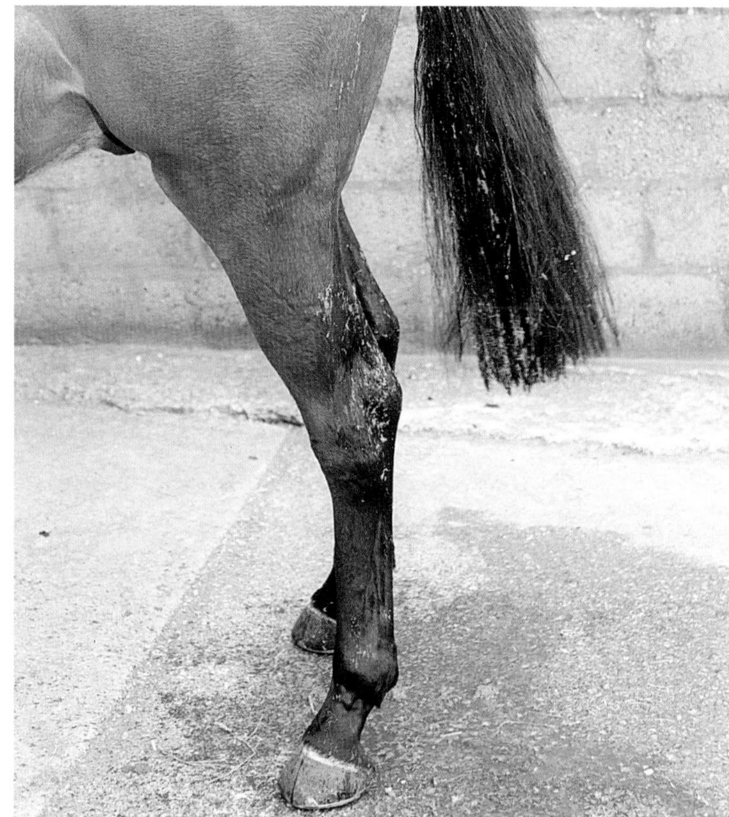

Diarrhoea can have serious consequences for the horse as it can very quickly lead to dehydration.

Breathing

Oxygen is supplied to the horse's body by way of the respiratory system. Air is drawn through the nose, past the larynx and into the windpipe (trachea), which is lined with rings of cartilage so that it does not collapse during normal breathing. The trachea passes into the thorax and into the lungs. At this point it branches into smaller and smaller tubes, known as bronchioles. At the end of the bronchioles are alveoli, through which carbon dioxide passes out of the body's system and oxygen passes into it. This system is highly developed to supply oxygen efficiently so that in the wild horses could run fast to escape from predators.

It is easy for small particles of debris to enter the respiratory system, but the cells lining the nasal passages, trachea and bronchi produce mucus, which helps to trap debris and airborne contaminants. There are small hair-like projections, known as cilia, to help move the contaminants out of the lungs and up the trachea so they can be coughed up. The principle respiratory problems the horse suffers are caused by obstructions of the airways due to infections and allergies, which create mucus and can provoke coughing.

For a diagram of the respiratory system, see page 11.

Quick-reference guide to ailments in this chapter:

Coughing

A cough is a reflex defence mechanism caused by mucus secretions or foreign bodies in the bronchi, trachea and larynx. The cough consists of three phases: a deep in-breath, a forced expiration of air against a closed glottis and a violent blast caused by the sudden opening of the glottis.

Symptoms Cough, possibly nasal discharge, difficulty breathing, heave lines and increased respiratory rate.

Causes Infectious and allergic respiratory conditions can create varying degrees of coughing. These include COPD, influenza, equine herpes, lungworm, viral pneumonia and choking.

Owner action Note whether the cough is, for example, harsh and dry or deep and moist. Offer feeds from the floor to encourage mucus to drain towards the head. Use dust-free bedding and make sure that the stable is well-ventilated. Consider soaking hay or provide a dust-free alternative. Turn the horse out as much as possible to reduce stable time.

DIAGNOSIS

This can be complicated and will involve an assessment of the other features of the condition together with listening to the heart, chest and trachea with a stethoscope and, possibly, examination of the nose, larynx and trachea with a fibre-optic endoscope. Samples of mucus and blood may be required to confirm clinical opinion. (See also specific conditions.)

Treatment Treatment depends on the condition causing the cough and will be dealt with in individual sections of this chapter.

Related conditions Choke (see page 43).

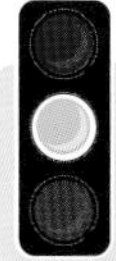

URGENCY INDICATOR

Fairly urgent. If in respiratory distress, very urgent.

COST

Fairly expensive, depending on diagnostic techniques and treatment. Bedding and feed may need to be changed to more expensive varieties.

Nasal discharge

Nasal discharges can be of mucus, blood, pus or food products. The underlying causes are excess mucus production resulting from allergic and infectious diseases or pus from abscesses, as in strangles or sinus infections. In cases of choke, it may be food mixed with saliva.

Symptoms Unilateral or bilateral nasal discharge. The discharge may be serous or thick, and may be smelly or contain blood.

Causes Upper or lower respiratory tract infections, guttural pouch problems, sinus problems, tooth root infections, allergies, choke, strangles and masses in the nasal chambers.

Owner action Nasal discharges indicate problems of the respiratory system. Seek early veterinary advice because of the possible number of potentially serious conditions that may cause the discharge. It is important for the diagnosis to note the nature of the discharge and whether it is from one or both nostrils.

DIAGNOSIS

Investigation as described for coughing will identify the cause. Endoscopy may be used to evaluate the respiratory tract. It may also be necessary to X-ray the head.

Treatment Treatment will depend on the underlying cause and will be covered in individual sections of this chapter.

WARNING Coughs and nasal discharges are often evidence of infectious diseases. Isolate any affected horses so that the condition does not spread.

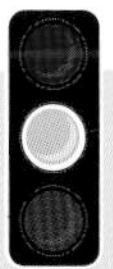

URGENCY INDICATOR

Fairly urgent. All coughs and nasal discharges should be investigated.

COST

Depends on the cause and diagnostic techniques used.

Respiratory distress

Diseases of the upper airway tend to cause difficulty breathing in; diseases of the lower lung tend to cause difficulty in breathing out. Some upper-airway obstructions are noticed only at fast exercise and usually cause an abnormal respiratory noise.

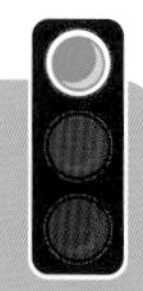

URGENCY INDICATOR

Urgent, because of the acute nature and rapid spread of these diseases and of the possible severe consequences if untreated.

COST

Low except in complicated cases.

The major respiratory diseases are equine influenza, equine herpes and equine viral arteritis. Many of the symptoms produced by these viral diseases are similar and lead to exercise intolerance, which results in fatigue when the horse is worked. Respiratory viral infections are more common in younger horses, particularly when they are stabled in groups.

Symptoms Loss of appetite, depression, coughing, loss of performance, raised temperature, sometimes swollen painful lymph nodes and nasal discharge, occasionally swelling of limbs and stiffness.

The symptoms of herpes tend to be less severe and the death rate lower than those resulting from influenza virus. Infection of pregnant mares with herpes EHV1 in the last third of pregnancy may cause abortion or the birth of weak foals. Neurological problems have also been seen after infection with herpes EHV1. Equine viral arteritis (EVA) is a severe disease in both young and old horses, and once infected some horses can stay infectious (carriers). It can also be transmitted venereally and therefore has major consequences for the breeding industry.

Causes Infections, viruses, bacteria, worms or allergies.

Owner action It is important to seek immediate veterinary advice.

Treatment Isolation and good nursing may be all that is required. Antibiotics can limit and prevent secondary infections, as can broncodilating drugs, which help to open up the bronchi to ease breathing. It is important that horses suffering from these viral infections are not stressed or exercised and are kept in a dust-free environment.

DIAGNOSIS

This involves a full clinical examination. Nasopharyngeal swabs, inserted up the nose to the back of the pharynx, may be taken for virus culture, and blood tests may be taken to identify viral infections. Often two blood samples taken 14 days apart will be required.

Related conditions Strangles (see page 55), lungworm (see page 46) and other conditions causing a nasal discharge or a cough, such as choke (see page 43).

Prevention New arrivals into an equine community should be isolated for three weeks and monitored for symptoms during that time. This is particularly important in non-vaccinated horses. Routine vaccination is extremely important and has done a great deal to reduce the occurrence of these diseases. Make sure that all stables, particularly those in barns, are properly ventilated. Avoid all contact between healthy and sick horses. Stop training and exercise to minimize stress. Isolate any horses with suspected or confirmed infection so that the problem does not spread to other animals.

Strangles

This common acute bacterial respiratory infection is most often seen in young animals, although it can occur at any age. It is highly contagious and can spread easily through a group of susceptible horses by either direct or indirect contact.

Symptoms The horse has a high temperature of 39.5–40.5°C (103–105°F). He will often be off his food, dull and lethargic. This is accompanied by a thick nasal discharge. Sometimes there is difficulty in swallowing and quite often an enlargement of the lymph glands under the jaw, which can soften and burst, discharging thick pus. Respiratory distress may be noted, and occasionally the infection can spread to other parts of the body and produce unusual symptoms (bastard strangles).

Cause Caused by the bacterium *Streptococcus equi*, which is very infectious.

Owner action Seek veterinary advice immediately and isolate the infected horse. Damp all feeds and offer only soft feed. Treat with a hot cloth and bathe any lymph node abscesses, but be careful not to let infected clothing come into contact with other horses. Isolate any horses that you suspect are infected.

Treatment Affected horses should be quarantined to contain the infection. Note that infected horses might still spread the disease many months after infection. Horses should remain in isolation for four to five weeks after symptoms have disappeared. Negative results from three culture swabs taken every seven to ten days are recommended before the horse is assumed clear of infection. Personal hygiene is extremely important when handling infectious cases. The bacteria are particularly sensitive to penicillin-type drugs, and if antibiotics are used the treatment must continue for several days after symptoms have disappeared. At-risk horses should have their temperatures taken daily and be treated as soon as any fever appears. Supportive therapy may be required in more severe cases.

DIAGNOSIS

A full clinical examination will be necessary. Naso-pharyngeal swabs, inserted up the nose to the back of the pharynx, or swabs from the abscess may be taken.

Related conditions Respiratory viral conditions (see page 54) and choke (see page 43).

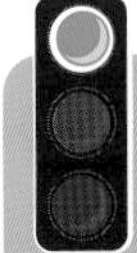

URGENCY INDICATOR

Urgent – seek veterinary advice immediately.

COST

Relatively inexpensive as long as early diagnosis is made.

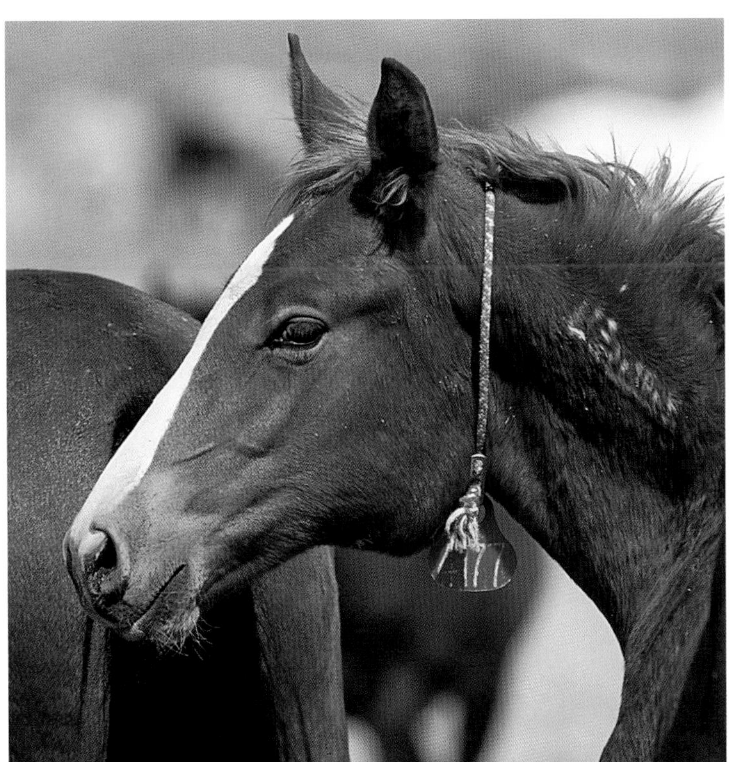

This foal with strangles displays the characteristic enlargement of the lymph glands associated with this infection.

Bacterial pneumonia

Pneumonia is an inflammation of the lung tissue, or inflammation of the airways. It can be caused by bacterial or viral agents.

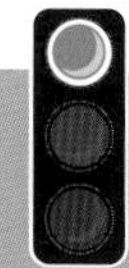

URGENCY INDICATOR

Very urgent. This acute disease can lead to severe lung damage and even death if not treated rapidly.

COST

Potentially expensive.

Symptoms Major symptoms are increased respiratory and heart rates accompanied by difficulty in breathing, nasal discharge, fever and coughing.

Causes There is often a history of exposure to stressful situations – such as transport, training, anaesthesia or, with foals, weaning – or the horse may have a previous history of viral tract infection, all of which can lead to depression of the immune system.

Owner action Requires immediate veterinary attention. Try to move the horse to a dust-free environment, ideally outside, or inside in a well-ventilated stable, with dust-free bedding and soaked hay.

DIAGNOSIS

This relies on a clinical examination. Endoscopy may be required and radiography and ultrasonography may be used to examine the chest cavity.

Treatment Depending on the severity of the condition, treatment will include antibiotics, anti-broncho-dilators and, possibly, the use of chest drains.

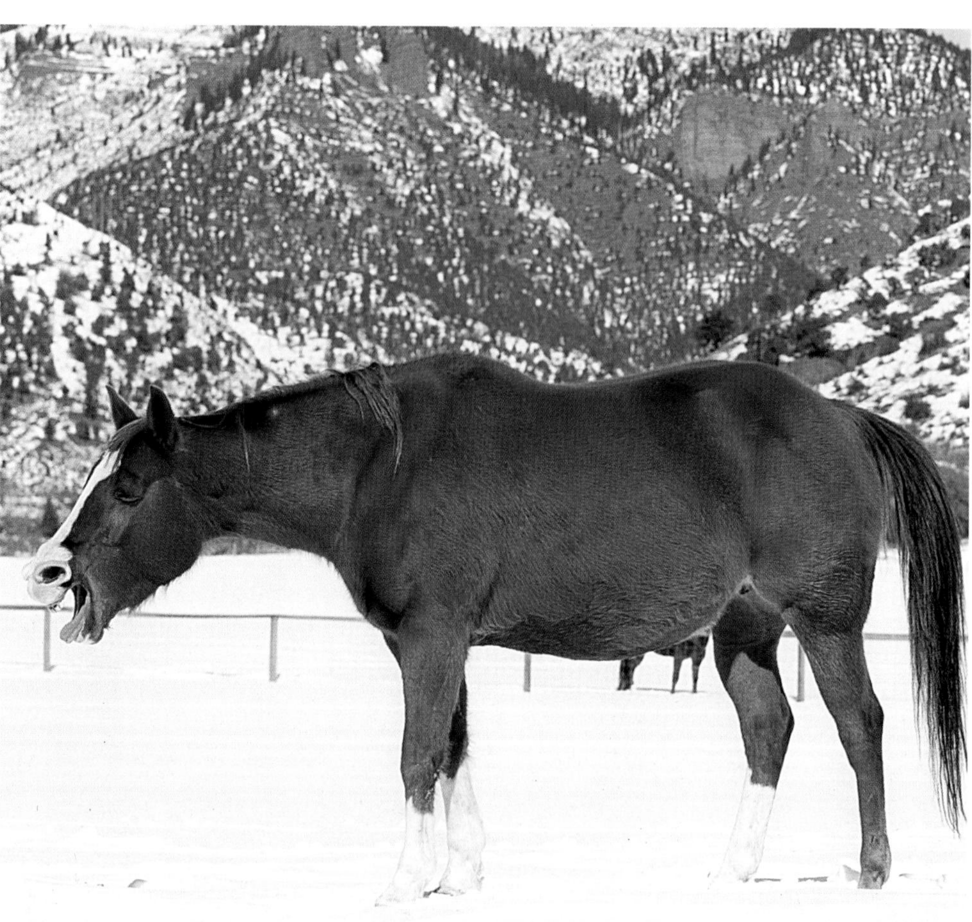

This horse is suffering from severe breathing difficulties and coughing, which could lead to major problems if not treated promptly.

Chronic obstructive pulmonary disease (COPD)

Also known as recurrent or reactive airway obstruction, this is one of the commonest diseases of the lower respiratory tract encountered in the UK. It is an allergic inflammation.

Symptoms Cough, nasal discharge and difficulty breathing.

Causes Spores and allergens collect in the bronchioles, causing an immune reaction and irritation. This can lead to increased mucus production in the small airways, which can eventually lead to obstruction of the small airways.

Owner action This problem requires immediate veterinary attention.

Treatment Treatment involves drugs to dilate the bronchioles and thin the mucus, and anti-inflammatories to decrease inflammation. These may be given orally, by injections or through inhalations. The treatment must also involve placing the horse in an environment where he is not exposed to the cause of the problem. For example, if it is spores and dust, the horse should be put outside or into a well-ventilated stable, with dust-free bedding, soaked hay or alternative feed sources. If the allergy is to pollen, a horse may need to be stabled or only put out at night. It is advisable to feed all food from the floor to aid in the drainage of mucus.

Related conditions Respiratory infections (see page 54).

DIAGNOSIS

This requires a full clinical examination. Endoscopy is commonly used to collect samples of the mucus and cells.

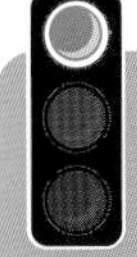

URGENCY INDICATOR

Urgent.

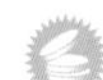

COST

Cost may increase with long-term treatment because COPD is likely to recur every year.

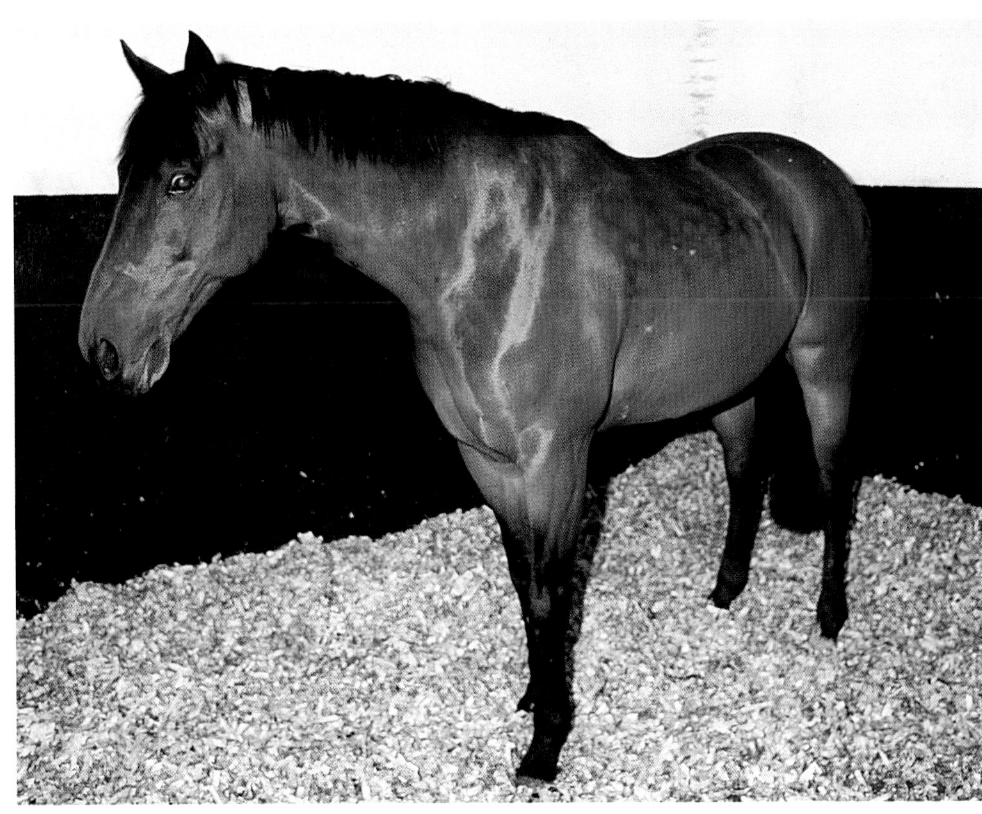

Dust-free bedding helps to produce a healthy environment for the horse.

Sinus problems

A sinus is basically a cavity in the skull, which is connected to the nasal cavity. The horse has two sinuses, the frontal sinus and the maxillary sinus, the latter also being split into two.

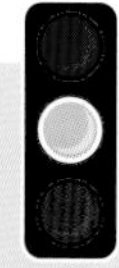

URGENCY INDICATOR

Fairly urgent to prevent further damage.

COST

Depends on the extent of the problem.

Symptoms Unilateral (from one nostril) nasal discharge.

Causes Bacterial infection of the sinuses. Because there is a close association between the teeth and the sinuses, the infection may involve the roots of the upper molar teeth.

Owner action As the symptoms are as for a possible infectious disease, isolate the horse and seek veterinary advice.

Treatment Treatment involves flushing the sinuses with an antibiotic and sometimes an antifungal mixture. Simple infections respond well to treatment.

DIAGNOSIS

Full clinical examination, and head X-rays showing the presence of fluid in the sinuses.

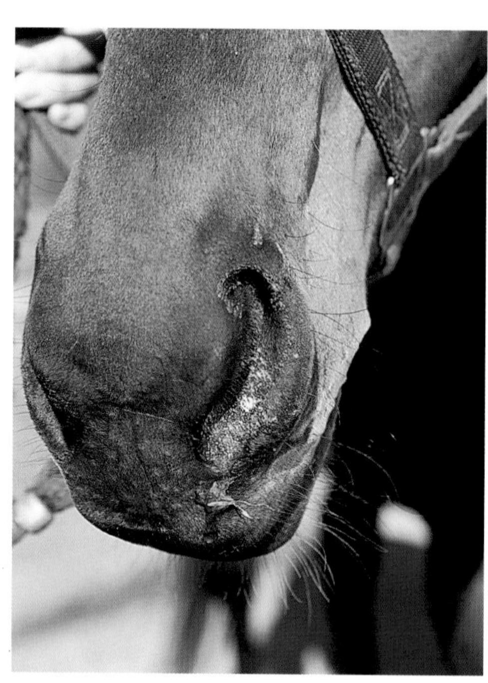

A persistant discharge from one nostril can indicate a guttural pouch disorder or an infection of the sinuses.

Nasal problems

The nasal cavity is the most proximal part of the respiratory tract. The nostrils are large, to enable the horse to breath as efficiently as possible, and lead to two openings: the upper false nostril, and the lower opening which leads into the nasal cavity.

Symptoms Nasal discharge, which may be bloody and smelly. Alterations in the airflow and respiratory noises.

Causes A number of problems can occur in the nasal passages, including infections, tumours and polyps.

Owner action As the symptoms are the same as for an infectious disease, the horse should be isolated in a dust-free environment and veterinary attention should be sought.

 **DIAGNOSIS**

Clinical examination, often using endoscopy and head X-rays.

Treatment This depends on the source of the problem but requires removal of the cause and treatment of any associated infection.

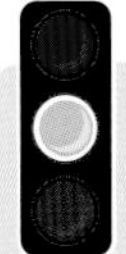

URGENCY INDICATOR

Fairly urgent to prevent further damage created by the infection.

 **COST**

Depends on the extent of the problem.

Guttural pouch disorders

The guttural pouch joins the pharynx through a slit-like orifice. The functions of this pouch are unclear, but because of its position several disorders with varying degrees of importance and severity may occur.

Symptoms A persistent nasal discharge from either one nostril or both, which may contain blood and be smelly. Swelling in the throat area. Unilateral facial paralysis and drooping of the eyelid.

Causes Bacterial or fungal infections that are localized in the guttural pouch.

Owner action This condition requires veterinary treatment as the symptoms are the same as for many respiratory tract infections. The horse should be isolated and fed from the floor to encourage nasal drainage.

Treatment This involves antibiotics, often in association with local irrigation to introduce antibiotics or fungicides directly into the guttural pouch.

 **DIAGNOSIS**

Clinical examination, and the use of endoscopy and/or head X-rays.

Related conditions Strangles (see page 55), sinusilis ethmoidal haematomas, tumours in the nasal cavities and upper respiratory tract infections.

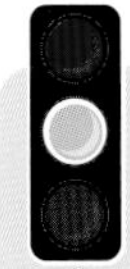

URGENCY INDICATOR

Fairly urgent.

 **COST**

Depends on diagnostic techniques, but likely to be fairly expensive.

Roaring

Roaring (idiopathic laryngeal hemiplegia) is an obstruction of the upper airways and causes a noise when the horse breathes in. It is usually first noticed in younger horses, particularly large thoroughbreds, in fast exercise. It more commonly affects the left-hand side of the larynx.

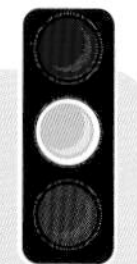

URGENCY INDICATOR

Fairly urgent in case there is a more sinister underlying cause.

 **COST**

Fairly expensive if treatment involves surgery.

Symptoms Loud roaring sound heard during exercise, coming from the upper respiratory tract and normally in the expiratory phase.

Causes Damage to the recurrent laryngeal nerves that control the muscles of the larynx.

Owner action If the horse's performance is poor or respiratory noise is evident, seek veterinary advice to ascertain the cause.

Treatment Surgical treatment is possible. In severe cases this involves surgery known as a 'tie back' operation (laryngoplasty). In less severe cases a 'hobday' procedure (ventrilectomy) is sufficient. The major problem with the 'tie back' operation is the possible complication of coughing caused by the inhalation of food after surgery.

 **DIAGNOSIS**

Upper airways obstructions may cause a respiratory noise, particularly during fast exercise. The condition is usually seen in thoroughbred horses and results in poor performance. It is visibly evident as wastage of the larynx muscles, which can be seen by examination with an endoscope.

Related conditions Soft palate displacement (see below), epiglottic cysts and other obstructions of the nasal passage, and diseases causing nasal deformity and obstruction – for example, sinusitis and tumour.

Soft palate dislocation

Another form of upper-airway obstruction, this is the dorsal displacement of the soft palate. The horse's soft palate is long and if it is displaced it can narrow the airways, causing difficulty with inhalation and exhalation and a gurgling noise during high-speed work.

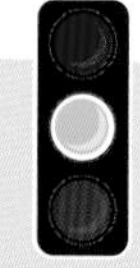

URGENCY INDICATOR

Fairly urgent.

 **COST**

Expensive if surgery is required.

Symptoms Difficulty breathing when exercising, often accompanied by a gurgling noise.

Causes The anatomy of the soft palate. The problem is usually noticed when a horse is tiring and the exertion requires maximum air intake.

Owner action Seek veterinary advice if any gurgling is heard.

Treatment In some cases the application of a tongue strap or straight bit will eliminate the problem. Various surgical procedures are used to sort out soft palate problems, but it is not clear how effective they are.

 **DIAGNOSIS**

The rider usually notices a gurgling noise during fast exercise and the horse may choke up, dramatically affecting his performance.

Related conditions Epiglottic entrapment, obstructions of the airways and roaring (see above).

Exercise-induced pulmonary haemorrhage (EIPH)

EIPH is a common disorder, particularly in thoroughbred and quarter horses, and it appears to be related to intense exercise. It occurs in a high percentage of young racehorses, but does not appear to affect their performance.

Symptoms Bleeding from the nose after intense exercise.

Causes Intense exercise, stress, low-grade respiratory disease.

Owner action Seek veterinary advice if a bloody discharge is noted issuing from the nostrils or the horse is exhibiting poor exercise-related performance.

Treatment Treatment involves rest and recovery of lung tissue and medication to treat any underlying lung disease. The diuretic drug furosemide is widely used in the USA before racing.

DIAGNOSIS

Needs to be confirmed by examination using an endoscope.

Related conditions Nasal tumours, nasal trauma and haemorrhage from the guttural pouches (see page 59).

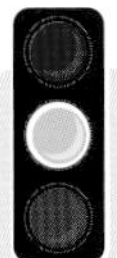

URGENCY INDICATOR

Urgent if a profuse and persistent haemorrhage from the nostrils occurs. Smaller bleeds, although not as urgent, should always be investigated.

COST

Inexpensive.

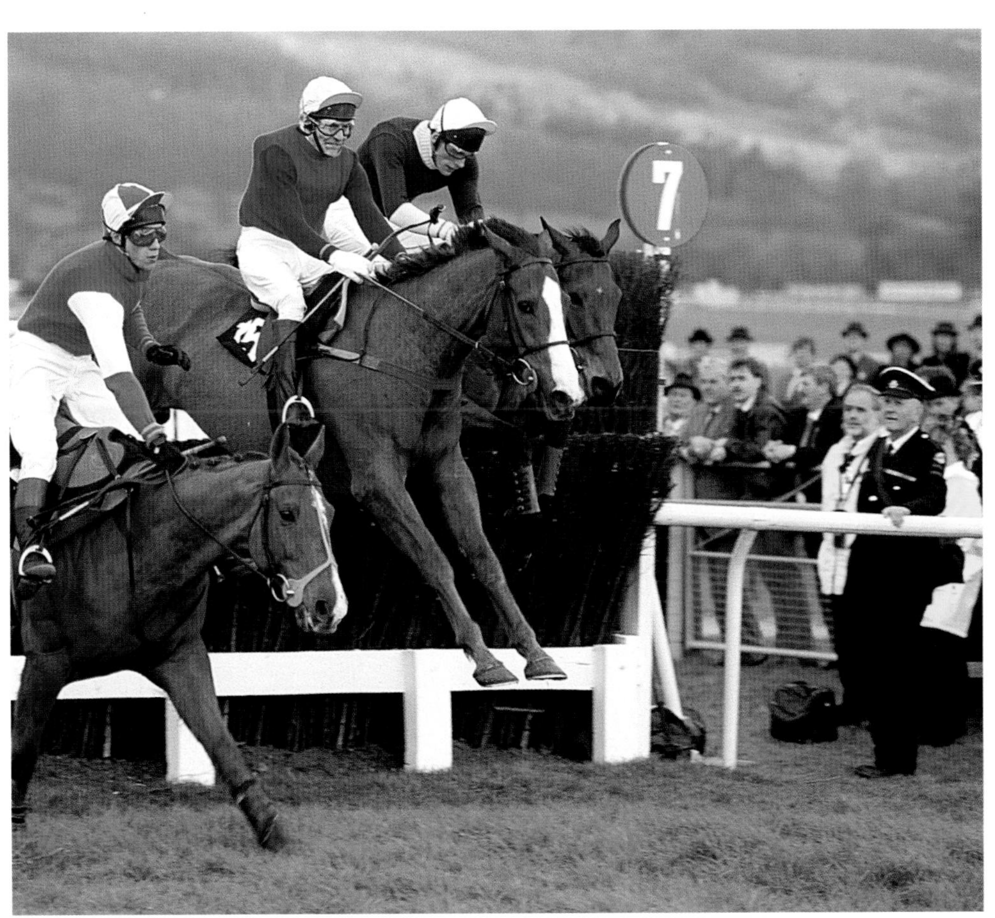

The stress of racing is a common cause of EIPH as it puts intense pressure on the lung tissue.

The heart

The horse's heart consists of four chambers – the right and left atriums and the right and left ventricles. The walls are made up of specialized muscle, which is electrically stimulated to contract, pumping blood through the heart. Valves between the chambers of the heart prevent the blood from flowing backwards when the chambers contract.

An electrocardiogram (ECG) is used to measure the electrical activity in the heart. It can show if there are any problems in conductivity, which may occur if there are changes in the muscle wall and is often heard as an arrhythmia (irregular heartbeat).

It is possible to hear four heart sounds with a stethoscope:

- closure of the atrio-ventricular valves, opening of the semi-lunar valves
- closure of the semi-lunar valves, opening of the atrio-ventricular valves
- end of rapid ventricular filling
- atrial systole

It is not always possible to hear the third and fourth heart sounds in a fit horse.

A heart murmur is heard when there is an abnormal flow of blood through the heart. It can be caused if valves leak and allow blood to flow back, by holes in the heart and by congenital problems (such as patent ductus aortus). Murmurs can also be heard if the viscosity of the blood changes, which happens, for example, in anaemia or hypoproteinaemia. Most heart murmurs are not significant, but it is always advisable to have them thoroughly checked by your vet because they may affect the riding potential of the horse.

Quick-reference guide to ailments in this chapter:

For **exercise intolerance**, see page 64

For **circulation problems**, see page 65

For **blood tests**, see pages 66–67

How the heart works

The heart is a large muscle that pumps blood to the lungs, where it collects oxygen, and then pumps the oxygenated blood around the body so that the cells in the body receive enough oxygen to function.

Measuring the horse's heart rate

A healthy horse has a regular heart rate of around 25–35 beats per minute, and it is quite easy to check this. The heart rate can be measured either by feeling the pulse under the horse's jaw or by placing your hand behind the left elbow and feeling for the apex heart beat. It is a good idea to find out your horse's heart rate when he is at rest, so that you have something to compare it against if problems arise in the future.

POSITION OF THE HEART

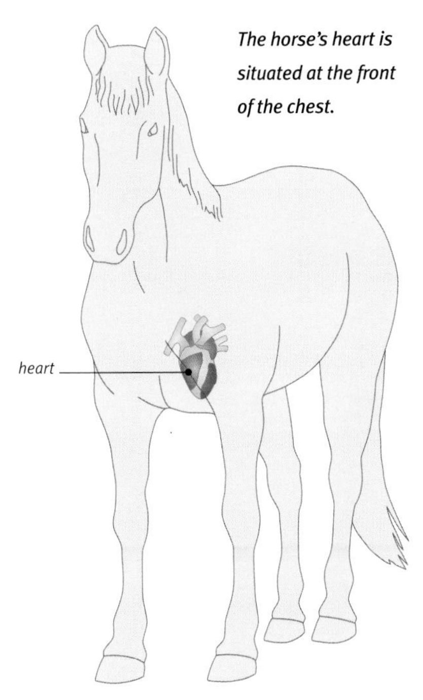

The horse's heart is situated at the front of the chest.

FLOW OF BLOOD IN THE HEART

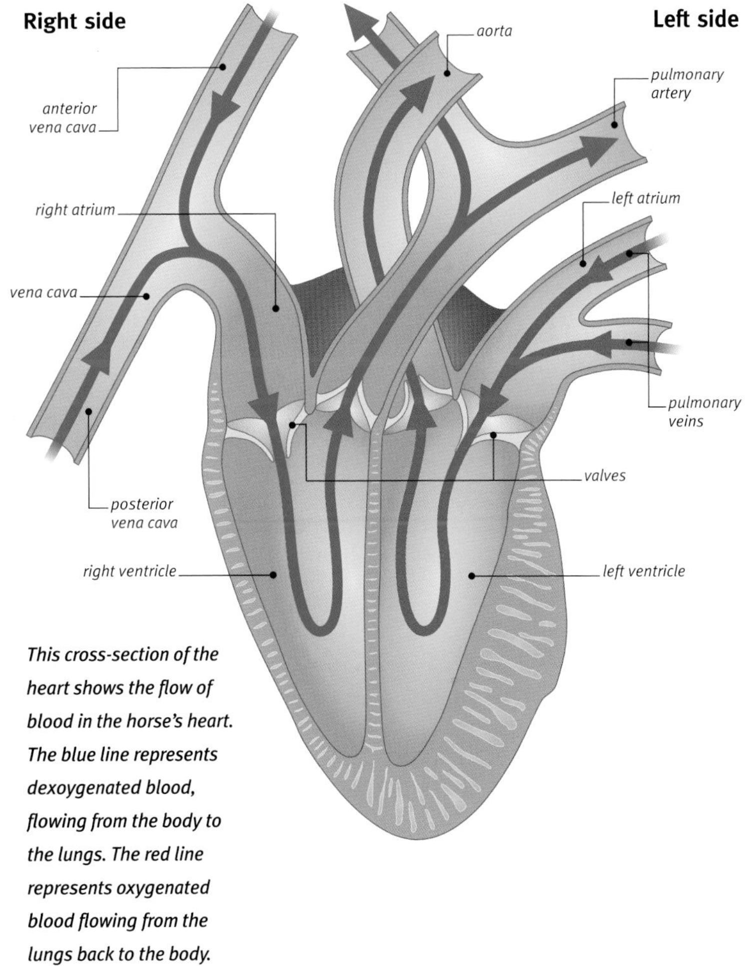

This cross-section of the heart shows the flow of blood in the horse's heart. The blue line represents dexoygenated blood, flowing from the body to the lungs. The red line represents oxygenated blood flowing from the lungs back to the body.

Exercise intolerance

This may only be evident in very active horses, and occurs when a horse starts to become abnormally tired and has a very slow recovery time after exercise. The horse will eventually refuse to go forward.

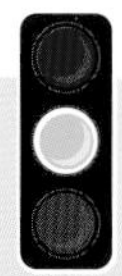

URGENCY INDICATOR

Fairly urgent.

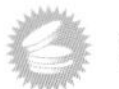

COST

Depends on the cause and treatments needed. The horse may be prevented from being ridden again.

Symptoms Loss of energy or slowing down – the horse becomes unusually tired after being worked or refuses to do work. Possible cough.

Causes Atrial fibrillation, pericarditis, myocardial disease, anaemia, viruses, infection, setfast, colic.

Owner action This condition will require veterinary investigation.

Treatment Treatment will depend on the cause. Some arrhythmias (irregular heartbeats) are treatable with drugs. Unfortunately, it is not yet possible to carry out open-heart surgery on horses, so other heart problems cannot be treated.

DIAGNOSIS

A full clinical examination is needed, both at rest and after exercise (if possible). The vet may also perform blood tests, cardiac auscultation (listening to the heart) and an ECG test.

It is often possible to keep affected horses as long as they are not ridden.

Related conditions Atrial fibrillation, pericarditis, myocardial disease, anaemia, viruses, infection, setfast (see page 78) and colic (see pages 44–45).

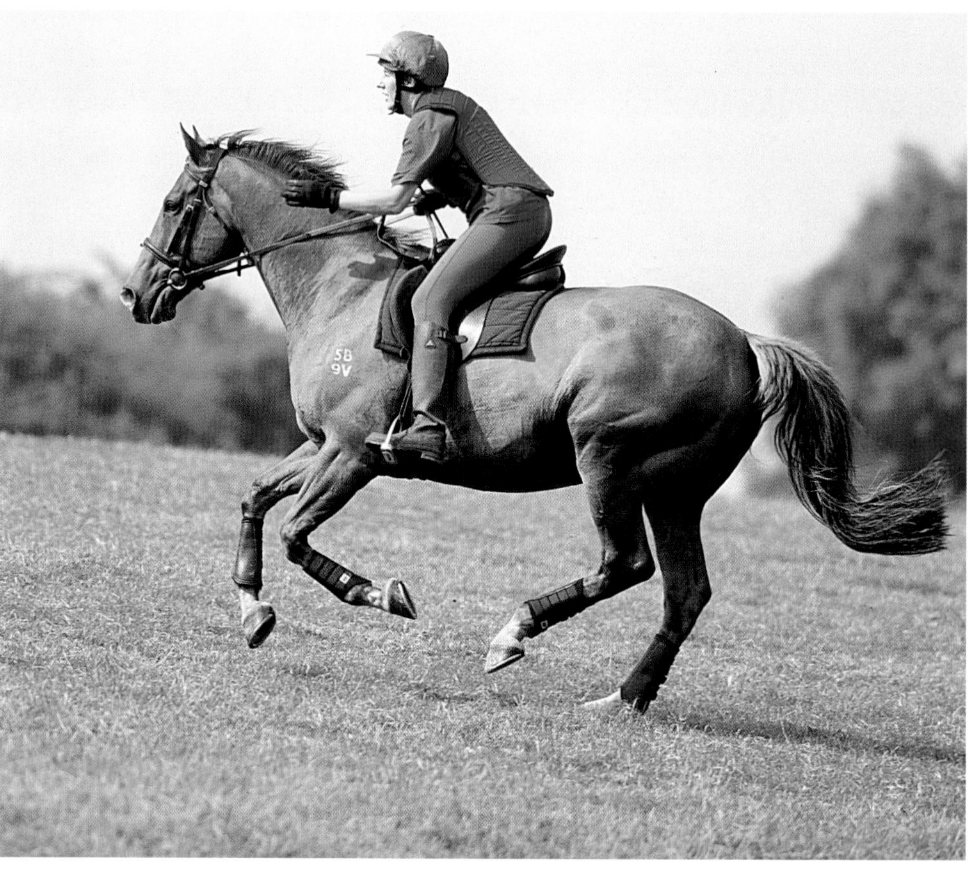

A fit and healthy horse should be able to carry a rider up slopes at speed without becoming abnormally tired and with a good recovery time.

Circulation problems

Abnormalities in the circulation of the blood can cause a number of different problems, such as oedema or thromboembolism.

Blood is carried from the heart in arteries, which branch off as they spread through the body into arterioles and then capillaries. Once the blood has been deoxygenated, it passes into veins to make its way back to the heart. (The only vein to contain oxygenated blood is the pulmonary vein.)

Arteries and arterioles are thick-walled vessels, lined with connective tissue and muscle, which carry blood under high pressure. Capillaries have very thin walls. Veins have slightly thicker walls, but also contain valves so that blood does not flow backwards. Blood vessels are not watertight. Fluid remains in the vessels through osmosis, the balance between the body and the blood. Any changes in the concentration of the blood, the speed of blood flow or inflammation of the vessels can cause leakage of fluid out of the vessels and into other tissue spaces (oedema).

OEDEMA

The leaking of fluid from vessels into other tissue spaces commonly occurs in the lungs (pulmonary oedema), abdomen (abdominal oedema), brain and cornea. Oedemas can also occur in the horse's legs, under the belly or under the chin.

Symptoms Fluid-filled limbs and swelling under the chin and belly. When the swelling is pressed in it leaves a dent.

Causes There are many causes of oedema; it is commonly seen in gastro-intestinal conditions that damage the tract, which results in the leakage of material into the body, affecting the concentration of the blood. A common cause of this is worms, and a horse with a heavy worm burden will often get oedema after it is wormed.

Any condition causing inflammation of the blood vessels, such as infections or wounds, will result in oedema. Heart conditions affecting the output or input pressure of the blood and allergic responses to bites or drugs can also cause oedema.

DIAGNOSIS

The following signs are used in the diagnosis of oedema: filled limbs and swelling under the chin and belly, which pits when pressed.

Owner action Hot and cold hosing can help to alleviate symptoms, as can exercise.

Treatment Treatment centres on improving the circulation. This will involve exercise, hot and cold hosing, and the use of steroids to help stabilize the damaged cells in the gastro-intestinal tract and prevent further damage. Diuretics may be used to reduce fluid retention.

OTHER CONDITIONS

Thromboembolism This is the blockage of arteries by clots. It can cause lameness (see pages 70–73) or collapsing on the hind limbs associated with patchy sweating. In extreme cases it can cause sudden death.

Lymphangitis Inflammation of the lymph vessels shows as severe, painful swelling in one limb (see page 77). Lymphangitis is not normally associated with infection.

URGENCY INDICATOR

Urgent.

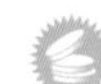

COST

Low, unless it becomes recurrent or requires prolonged treatment.

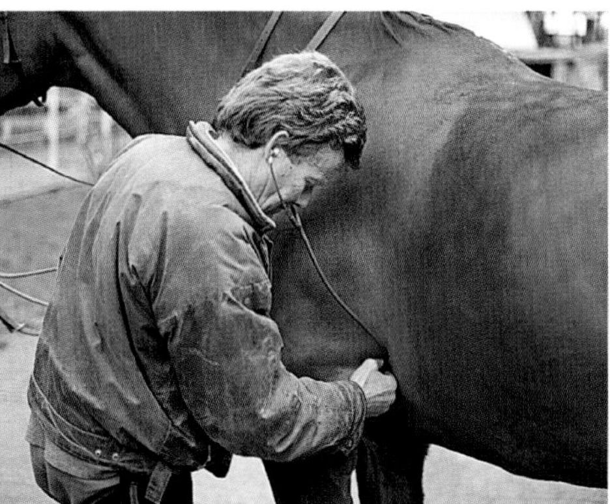

Listening to the heart beat with a stethoscope is one of the first tests that a vet will perform when diagnosing possible heart and circulatory problems.

Understanding blood tests

Blood tests analyse the two main components of the blood: the cells and their environment. Blood may be taken to test for specific viruses. It can also be cultured for bacteria and examined for blood-borne parasites. The main terms involved in blood testing are explained here so that you will be better placed to understand the results of any tests carried out on your horse.

HAEMATOLOGY

This is the study of the physiology of the blood. It is used to investigate blood cells and their haemoglobin levels.

Haematocrit (HCT) or packed cell volume (PCV)

The number of red blood cells is used in the diagnosis of anaemia and dehydration. Anaemia, which occurs when there is a drop in the PCV, has many causes, and symptoms include pale mucous membranes, lethargy and exercise intolerance.

Haemoglobin (HGB)

Haemoglobin is the protein in red blood cells that carries oxygen. Competing horses require a high level of haemoglobin in their blood to allow them to work as efficiently as possible. Low haemoglobin levels are associated with anaemia, among other disorders.

Mean corpuscular haemoglobin concentration (MCHC)

Establishing the average amount of haemoglobin in a cell makes it possible to distinguish low haemoglobin resulting from too few red blood cells from red blood cells that do not produce sufficient haemoglobin.

White blood cells (WBC)

White cells fight infection, but abnormally high WBC counts can also indicate leukaemia. The WBC count is a combined count of the different types of WBC: granulocytes and lymphocytes.

Viewed under the microscope, granulocytes have a granular appearance. There are three different types:

- **Neutrophils** are cells that eat and break down foreign agents, such as bacteria. It is possible to date these cells, which helps to determine how recent an infection is. Their numbers become elevated in response to inflammation, such as after a wound.
- **Eosinophils** are mainly involved with infections involving parasites, such as worms, and they can also be elevated in response to specific conditions, such as allergies.
- **Basophils** are involved to a lesser degree than the other two types of granulocytes in response to inflammation and parasites.

Lymphocytes are small cells, whose numbers are often elevated in viral infections. There are two main types:

- **Platelets** (PLT) are involved in clotting; low numbers can indicate clotting problems.
- **Reticulocytes** are immature red blood cells. Numbers become elevated when the body is trying to regenerate red blood cells, such as after blood loss.

BIOCHEMISTRY

Biochemisty is the study of the enzymes and ions normally carried in the blood and determines levels of minerals, salts and proteins.

Albumin

This protein is synthesized by the liver and carried principally in red blood cells. Low albumin can occur if the number of red blood cells is reduced, if levels produced by the liver decline or if there is excessive loss in the urine or gastro-intestinal system. Increased albumin occurs in dehydration.

Bile acids

These acids are synthesized in the liver and are an indicator of liver function.

Creatinine

This nitrogenous compound is formed in the muscle and passed out in the urine. Levels are elevated after muscle damage, such as in setfast, or kidney failure.

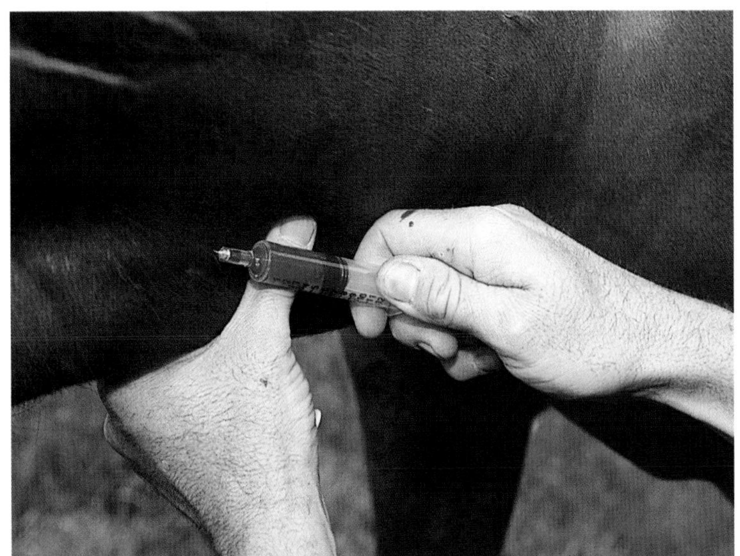

Taking a blood sample from the horse's jugular artery.

Glucobulins

These proteins are found in blood plasma and are involved in a range of activities, including the production of antibodies, fighting inflammation and clotting. They are formed from a number of different enzymes:

- **Alkaline phosphatase** (ALP) is found in cell membranes, and levels are elevated in liver, bone and intestinal problems.
- **Aspartate aminotransferase** (AST) is found in skeletal and cardiac muscle and in the liver. If any of these structures is damaged or inflamed, AST leaks into the blood stream.
- **Creatinine phosphokinase** (CK) is found in skeletal and cardiac muscle and in brain tissue; levels become elevated if any of these tissues is damaged.
- **Gamma glutamyl transferase** (GGT) levels become elevated in liver, kidney or pancreatic diseases. Horses rarely suffer from diseases of the kidney and pancreas, so this is a useful indicator of liver problems.
- **Glutamate dehydrogenase** (GLDH) levels become elevated only as a result of damage to the liver.
- **Lactate dehydrogenase** (LDH) is found in many tissues, including the liver, intestine, skeletal muscle, kidney and heart, and levels become elevated if any of these tissues are damaged.

Glucose

Elevated glucose levels are common in horses that are stressed, pregnant and obese, and in Shetland ponies. They can also become elevated in Cushing's disease (see page 27).

Urea

This is formed in the liver and filtered out of the blood in the kidneys. Blood levels become elevated in kidney disease, but small increases are also seen in horses that are dehydrated or that are fed on high-protein diets.

Lameness and traumatic injury

The horse is a supremely developed athlete. As a prey animal, he evolved with the ability to outpace predators with sudden and maintainable bursts of speed. Over many thousands of years this led to the development of the horse we know today. Selective breeding by humans has been partly responsible for the widely varying physiques and abilities of the different breeds of horses, but whether we are looking at the child's pony or the winning racehorse, the principles that have developed their relative athleticism are the same.

The horse's specialized locomotive system consists of muscles, bones, joints, tendons and ligaments, all of which are controlled by the central nervous system. Contact with the ground is through the horse's foot, which has evolved to absorb concussion and to support the weight of the body. Motion is produced by the pull of the large muscle masses, attached by means of a complicated system of tendons to the bones of the lower limbs, causing leverage and movement. The co-ordination between the muscles, tendons and ligaments is made possible by an enormously complex system, which also allows the limbs to remain stable and the horse to sleep standing up.

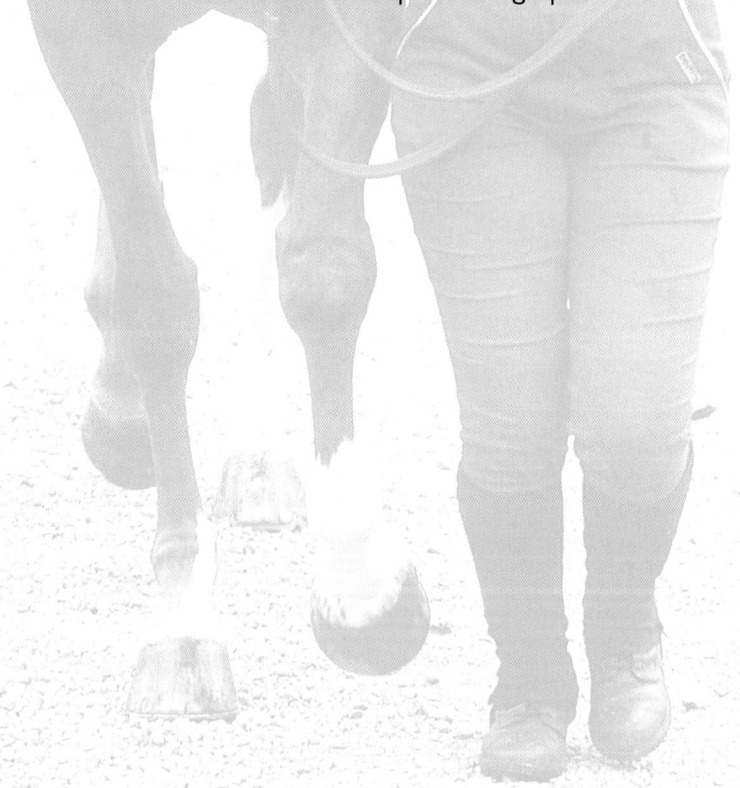

Quick-reference guide to ailments in this chapter:

The foot

The foot is a highly evolved part of the body, which supports the weight of the horse. Many forces work on the foot, and in a sound horse these work in equilibrium. However, when one force changes or the sole of the foot becomes painful, the balance is lost and the horse becomes lame.

The hoof is a structure that knits to the pedal bone by multiple, finger-like projections, called laminae. Both the pedal bone and the hoof have a set of laminae, which spread the force of the body and support the pedal bone. There are over 60,000 laminae attachments in the hoof, which equates to about 2.5sq m (8sq ft) of area for the attachment of hoof to bone – that is, about 125g (4oz) per 2.5 sq cm (1 sq in) of attachment when the animal is supporting its entire weight on one foot.

The pedal bone is the small triangular bone that mirrors the hoof wall and lies within the hoof surrounded by the laminae.

THE HOOF

The sole of the horse's foot.

THE FOOT

A cross-section of the horse's lower leg and foot.

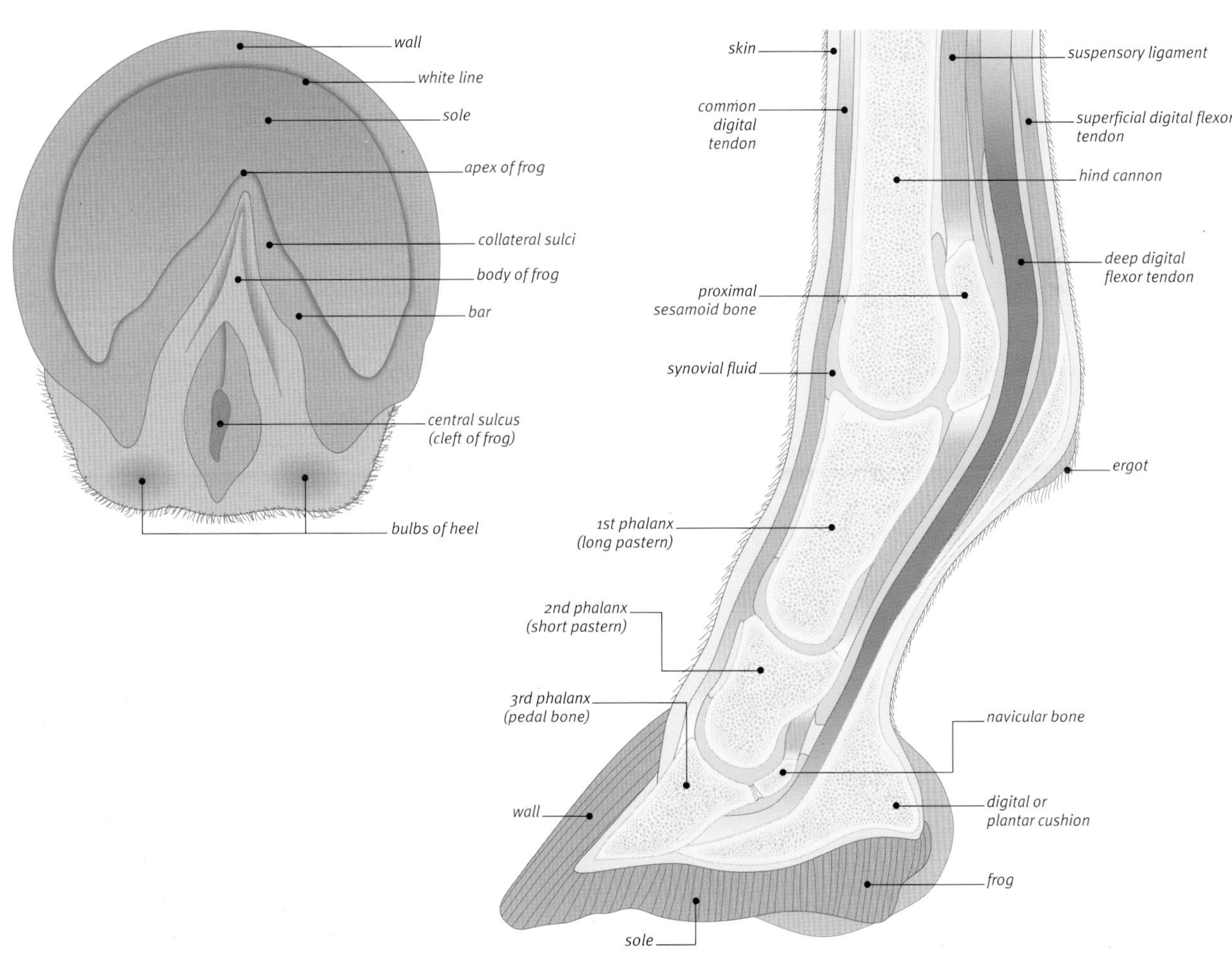

Investigating lameness

An examination will determine whether the horse is lame and which leg is affected. It will also identify the part of the leg that is affected and what is causing the problem. The significance of the problem, the treatment required and, indeed, the horse's future will be assessed.

The examination will also include observation of the horse's stance and whether any limb is rested to reduce weight bearing. Muscle wastage can be a useful indicator if the horse has been lame for some time.

Case history

The horse's recent history and performance record are noted and assessed and any recent changes recorded.

Trotting up

The horse is normally trotted in a straight line on a firm, non-slip surface so that the movement of the head as he approaches the observer and the movement of the hindquarters as he moves away can be noted. On a second trot-up the action of the individual limbs is observed. The horse is also usually turned tightly in a circle in both directions and backed by four or five strides. These movements are usually sufficient for the vet to make a decision about the lame limb or limbs.

Indicators of lameness during the trot-up include loss of symmetry of the stride and abnormal movements of the head. If the lameness is of a front limb the head will tend to 'go down' as the sound front foot comes to the ground and 'go up' as the lame foot comes to the ground. If a back leg is lame there will be a hike of the hip on the lame side.

Performing a flexion test to see whether the horse has a sprain.

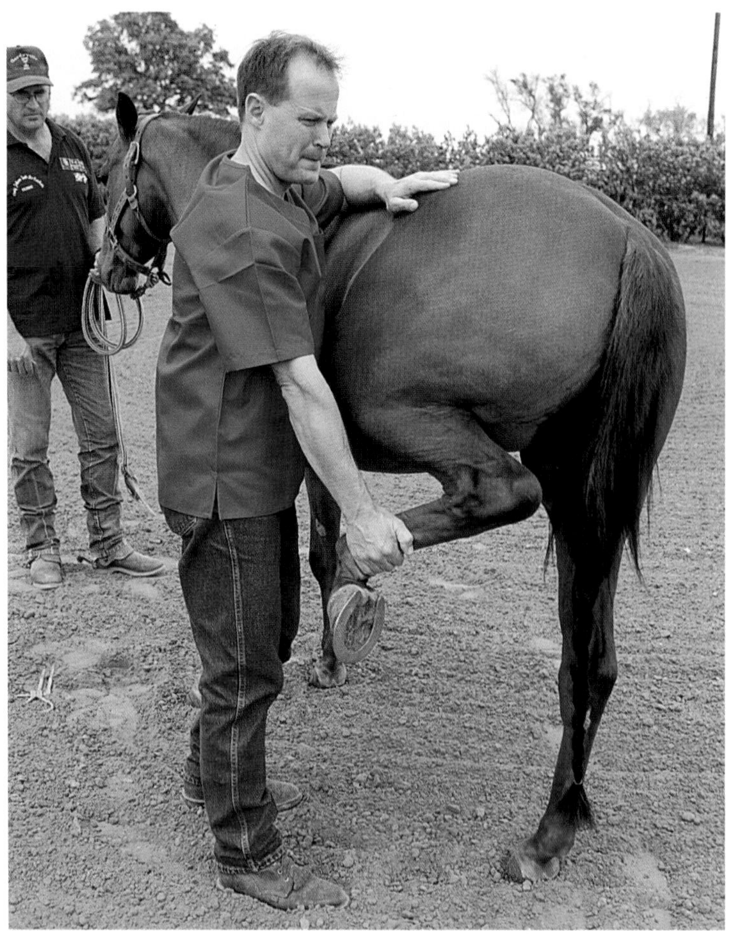

Lungeing

This is invaluable in detecting lameness, which will increase or decrease depending on the rein on which the horse is lunged.

Flexion and extension tests

This involves the horse's leg being held in flexion or extension for approximately 60 seconds, after which the horse is re-trotted and re-assessed. These tests help to identify the joints that are causing the lameness and are particularly useful if the problem is slight.

Clinical examination

After the preliminary examination to assess which limb or limbs are involved, a detailed physical examination will be made to identify any alterations in shape or any swelling. The vet will examine for pain by pressure and palpation and for restrictive movement with crepitus (crunching of the joint bones) and heat. The use of hoof testers is essential because a high percentage of lameness is in the foot.

Nerve and joint blocks

If there is no obvious site of lameness, diagnostic nerve blocks can help. Local anaesthetic is used to freeze the limb, usually from the bottom upwards, to isolate the source of the lameness. When the painful area is locally anaesthetized the horse will be able to walk normally. Similarly, the use of local anaesthetic injected into joints is a useful diagnostic aid.

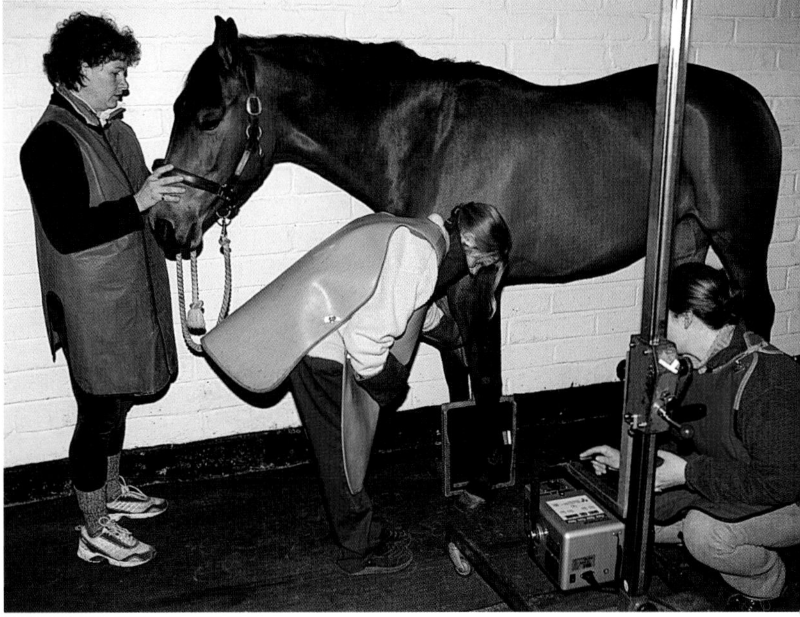

X-rays will enable the vet to see if there is a fracture or any other changes in the bone structure.

Further examination

X-rays may be necessary to detect bony changes. Ultrasonic diagnosis is useful for identifying soft tissue changes, particularly in the tendons and ligaments. Nowadays more sophisticated techniques are necessary for complicated cases and involve bone scanning (scintigraphy) and magnetic resonance imaging (MRI). Arthroscopy. which makes it possible to look inside joint cavities, is sometimes also used.

PEDAL OSTITIS

This condition is inflammation of the pedal bone and is caused by trauma to the bone by the action of the horse. Although pedal ostitis is rare, it involves changes in the nature of the bone and is best diagnosed by nerve block and X-ray. Care must be taken in diagnosis, because the margins of the pedal bone are remodelled throughout the life of a high percentage of sound horses.

Treatment Anti-inflammatories and antibiotics should be given. Often the infected bone is removed and antibiotics are put directly into the bone. Treatment will often take a long time, and require repeated procedures.

FRACTURE OF THE PEDAL BONE

The pedal bone may fracture in a number of places, the most common being the extensor process, where there are tendonous attachments to the top and front of the pedal bone. Fractures through the body of the pedal bone can occur at any site and present more of a problem if they involve the articular surface.

Treatment The hoof wall acts as a splint for the pedal bone. In simple cases not involving the articular surface, fitting with a special shoe may be all that is required. However, if the articular surface is involved surgical repair will be necessary.

SIDE BONES

Side bones occur when the lateral cartilages within the hoof become bony (a process called ossification). They are a common response to the shod horse working on a hard surface. As long as they are not associated with any joint changes and the conformation of the foot allows room for side bone development, lameness is usually seen only during the formation of the side bone. Side bones in horses with poor conformation can create permanent or intermittent lameness.

Treatment Treatment is not usually required.

Lower limb lameness

Lower limb lameness is that which is associated with the horse's foot. The principle causes of such lameness are explained here.

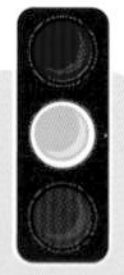

URGENCY INDICATOR

Fairly urgent. The sooner lameness is diagnosed and treated, the better the prognosis.

 **COST**

Usually low.

Symptoms Lameness, which may be intermittent and, if mild, obvious only when the horse moves in tight circles. Other symptoms are increased strength of the digital artery pulse, heat in the foot, stumbling, reluctance to move and lameness on hard surfaces.

Causes Navicular syndrome, laminitis, bruising, corns, seedy toe, thrush, tumours, abscesses, osteomylitis, shoeing lameness.

Owner action Rest the horse and seek veterinary advice. If an abscess is suspected the foot may be poulticed or tubbed.

 **DIAGNOSIS**

This will require an examination (see pages 70–71) and probably the use of nerve blocks to isolate the pain. The foot will be thoroughly examined and the shoes may be removed. X-rays may be required.

Treatment Depends on the cause; see separate conditions below.

NAVICULAR SYNDROME

This condition, which causes pain in the navicular bone, has many causes, including poor blood flow to the navicular bone, repeated stress leading to inflammation, infection and trauma. It tends to affect front feet and commonly shows as intermittent lameness, which may be obvious only when the horse moves in a tight circle. The horse often stumbles and may point his feet forward when standing and move his bedding around to support the heel.

Treatment No single treatment is wholly successful. A combination of anti-inflammatories and drugs to decrease the pressure of the blood in the feet is usually combined with shoeing and foot trimming to alleviate pressure on the heels.

BRUISED SOLE

Flat-footed, thin-soled horses are susceptible to solar bruising after contact with solid objects or work on hard, stony ground.

Treatment Rest and anti-inflammatories. If the sole has been punctured, the foot should be poulticed and may require antibiotics.

SEEDY TOE

Also known as white line, seedy toe occurs where the hoof separates along the white line of the sole. Dirt and grit get into the gap and can cause abscesses. It may be caused by a fungal infection.

Treatment The separated part of the hoof is removed. The foot may need to be poulticed or soaked in fungicides.

CORNS

A corn is a bruise that occurs between the wall and the bar of the foot. It is often caused by ill-fitting shoes.

Treatment Corns can often be pared by the vet or farrier. The foot should be trimmed correctly and the shoes refitted.

THRUSH

This fungal condition of the frog occurs in warm, moist conditions and is common in boxed horses, with inadequate or dirty bedding. Horses with a long toe or contracted heels tend to develop a deep frog cleft, making them susceptible to this condition.

Treatment Regular cleaning of the feet and bathing in antiseptic solutions. The foot should be dried afterwards.

SHOEING LAMENESS

Nail bind is caused if nails are placed too close to the sensitive white line. This is very painful and often requires the shoe to be removed. Nail prick occurs if a nail pierces the white line, introducing infection. The horse will resent the nail being placed and, when it is removed, it will often bleed.

Treatment Soaking the foot in disinfectant normally prevents infection, but antibiotics may be required.

SOLAR ABSCESSES AND OSTEOMYLITIS

Both conditions are caused by pieces of grit working through the sole. The pressure of the pus on the sensitive structures of the foot is very painful. If severe or left untreated, the pedal bone can become infected.

Treatment Treatment for abscesses involves poulticing the foot and releasing the pus. The vet or farrier may be unable to find the pus at first, but poulticing encourages the pus to track towards the sole and it can often be found in two to three days. If the pus is deep within the hoof it may burst out at the coronary band. Antibiotics may be given once the abscess has been drained.

Osteomylitis is diagnosed by X-ray, and treatment involves removing the infected bone under an anaesthetic.

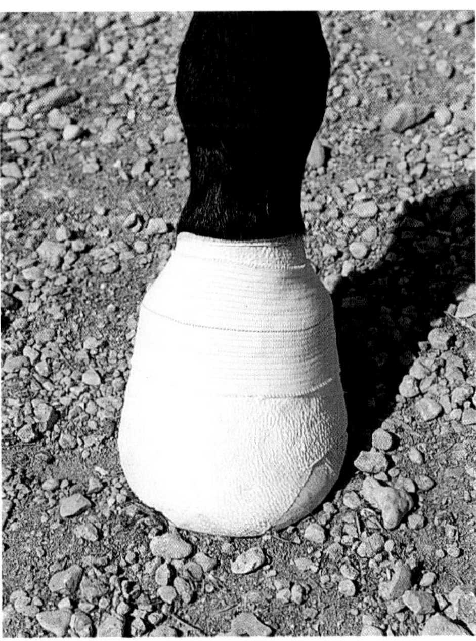

A poultice can be applied to the hoof to help draw pus out from a solar abscess.

Laminitis

Laminitis, commonest in ponies and unfit horses, is the inflammation of the laminae in the foot, and severe cases cause the structure of the laminae to pull apart. It can result in the pedal bone rotating from the force of the deep digital flexor tendon pulling it backwards; this is called rotation.

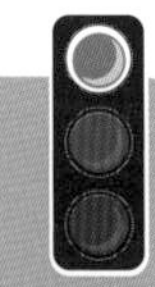

URGENCY INDICATOR

Urgent. The longer it is left, the more difficult the condition is to treat and the more irreversible the changes in the foot.

COST

Relatively cheap if not accompanied by pedal bone rotation and responds to treatment in two or three days. Expensive and long term if it does not respond well to treatment or already involves changes to the pedal bone.

Symptoms These depend on the severity of the condition but include a shifting gait at rest, reluctance to move, walking with a heel-first stance and lying down.

Causes Carbohydrate overload, toxaemia or septicaemia, concussion and mechanical overload, exogenous cortico-steroids, Cushing's disease, liver dysfunction, hypothyroidism, allergic reaction, high-pasture oestrogen and insulin resistance.

Owner action Gradually stop all hard feed and give hay or a similar fibre-only food. Box rest on deep bedding. Call the vet to examine and treat the horse.

Treatment Stop all hard feed. Box rest on deep bedding. Anti-inflammatories and analgesics will be used, and drugs may be used to relax the vessels in the hoof to help reduce inflammation. Feed may be supplemented to improve hoof condition and help reduce inflammation; MSM and Methione are examples. Frog supports are often used, as well as foot trimming and surgical shoeing.

DIAGNOSIS

Diagnosis is made from the following symptoms: reluctance to walk, increased digital pulses in the foot (often accompanied by heat in the hoofs), walking and standing predominantly on the heels, pain on hoof testers over the front of the foot. Radiography may be used to examine the foot.

Related conditions Colic (see pages 44–45), solar bruising or abscess (see pages 72–73).

This diagram shows the displacement of the foot caused by laminitis. The red outline indicates the position of the foot bones in a horse with laminitis.

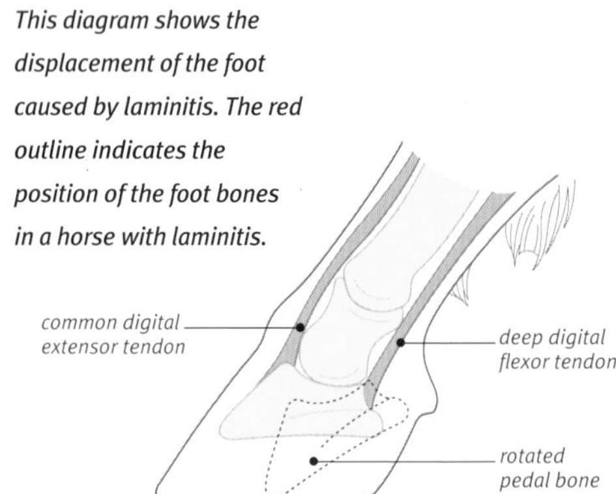

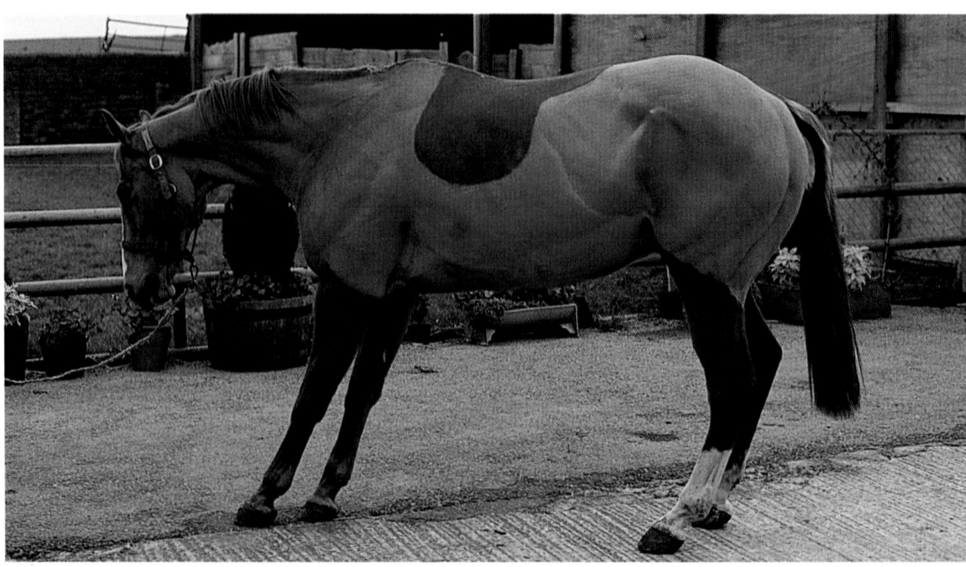

This stance is typical of a horse suffering from laminitis.

Degenerate joint disease (DJD)

Degenerate joint disease (DJD) is an extremely complicated subject, which is still poorly understood, but it is basically a wear-and-tear injury of the joints.

Symptoms Lameness or heat and swelling of the joints.

Causes Stress on the joint is often seen in a horse that has had an active competition life. Age, nutrition and genetic make-up also play a part. Competitive minor trauma is probably the most important contributory factor.

Owner action If you notice heat and swelling of the joints or lameness, seek veterinary advice.

Treatment Unfortunately, this condition cannot be cured once established. However, treatments can help to alleviate the symptoms and prolong the working life. Initially, rest is vital to allow the inflammation to settle down. Anti-inflammatories, both non-steroidal anti-inflammatories (NSAIDs) and corticosteroids, are of use. Steroids must be used with great care and the horse must not be returned to work too early on non-steroidal anti-inflammatories as these will mask any pain. Medication such as hyaluronic acid, glycosaminoglycanpolyphosphate and cartrophen have been shown to improve joint function. Procedures such as arthroscopy can also be useful but are expensive.

Related conditions Local trauma and strains.

DIAGNOSIS

Diagnosis is usually made by clinical examination. This may include flexion tests and the use of local anaesthetic injected into the joint followed by X-rays and possible scans of the joint.

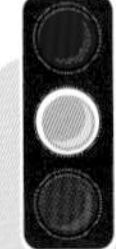

URGENCY INDICATOR

Fairly urgent. This type of joint disease is usually slowly progressive, but the earlier it is treated the better.

COST

Ongoing costs could be high.

Joint injuries

Any wound over or close to a joint is potentially very serious, especially if it penetrates into the joint itself.

Symptoms These are usually pain and lameness, but the penetration can be quite small and appear insignificant.

Causes Penetration of the joint by some kind of foreign body.

Owner action Call out the vet immediately. The wound must be examined and treated as quickly as possible.

Treatment If a joint has been penetrated, it will need to be flushed out with an antibiotic.

Related conditions Sprain and DJD (see above).

DIAGNOSIS

It is extremely important to establish whether the penetration is into the joint. Synovial fluid may be seen leaking from the joint, but the diagnosis can be more difficult and must be made with X-rays or ultrasound. Often the joint is filled with sterile saline under pressure – if there is communication with the joint, then fluid will flow through the wound.

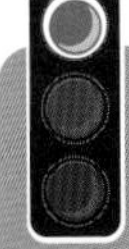

URGENCY INDICATOR

Urgent. Any penetrative wound close to a joint should be considered an emergency.

COST

High.

Tendon injuries

Tendons are made up of stands of collagen fibre, and the strength of the tissues derives from collective alignment. Tendon strains tear the fibres, leading to rupture and destruction of the fibre pattern.

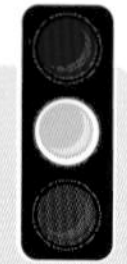

URGENCY INDICATOR

Fairly urgent. Heat or pain or other symptoms of inflammation in the leg must be investigated at an early stage to prevent further tendon damage.

 **COST**

The major cost is the long period of rehabilitation.

Tendon injuries commonly occur in the deep and superficial flexor tendons in the area between the knee and the fetlock, but occasionally also below the fetlock.

Symptoms Variable degree of lameness, with swelling and heat in the tendon.

Causes Increased pressure-loading on the tendons often creates tendon strain when the muscles of galloping horses begin to tire.

Owner action Heat and pain in the tendon area should always be investigated, even if the horse is not lame.

Treatment There have probably been more treatments for tendon conditions than any other musculo-skeletal problem. Initial treatment should be aimed at reducing inflammation and usually involves cold treatment and bandage support. Cold hosing combined with the careful application of ice (beware of frostbite) are the best methods. Support bandaging should be continued, and anti-inflammatory products are useful initially to reduce the haemorrhage and swelling. All tendon injuries require long periods of rest and rehabilitation. Other treatment techniques involve tendon splitting, tendon injections, carbon fibre implants and thermo-quartery. Superior check ligament desmotomy has in some cases proved to be useful.

Despite the various treatments used there is a high rate of recurrence, and no matter what treatment is used, a long period of rehabilitation will be necessary.

 **DIAGNOSIS**

Diagnosis can be confirmed and the degree of damage assessed by ultrasonic scanning.

Related conditions Suspensory strains (see page 77) and other conditions of the tendon, such as tendon sheath infections.

WARNING In the early stages there may be little clinical evidence, so if tendon injury is suspected treatment should be undertaken immediately.

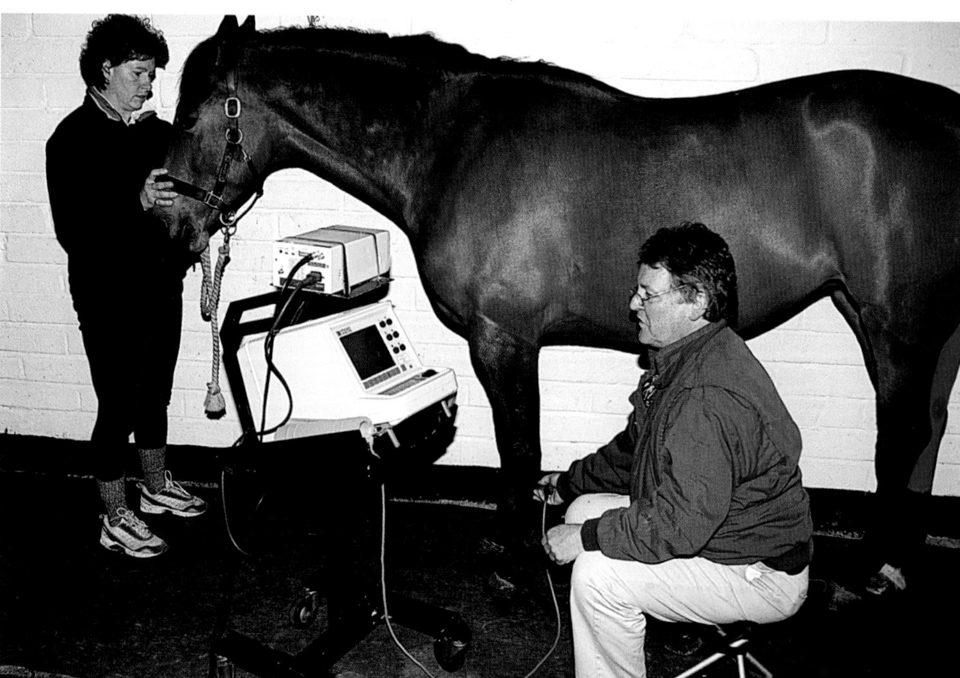

Ultrasonic scanning can be used to confirm both the diagnosis and extent of a tendon injury.

Suspensory strains

The suspensory ligaments are part of the stay apparatus, a mechanism consisting of ligaments, tendons and muscles. They attach the back of the cannon bone to the sesamoid bones and insert into the pastern and pedal bone. Inflammation of this ligament is known as a desmitis.

Symptoms Lameness or pain and swelling in the sesamoid ligaments.

Causes Unequal loading of the fetlock joint while it is extended, so that one side bears more strain than the other. Lack of co-ordination brought on by fatigue in the performance horse and poor conformation and shoeing may lead to the problem.

Owner action Seek veterinary advice about swelling or pain in the sesamoid ligaments. In the meantime, the horse should be rested and cold treatment given.

Treatment The success of treatment depends on the site of the strain. Single-branch strains, particularly from the middle of the branch, are likely to recover best. Tears at the attachment to the bones are likely to be a long-term problem.

DIAGNOSIS

This is made on the clinical signs and can be confirmed by nerve block. X-rays may be needed to rule out fracture of the sesamoid bone, and ultrasonic scanning can be used to ascertain the extent of the damage.

Primary treatments are the application of firm pressure bandages and cold treatment with immobilization and box rest, but healing is lengthy and can take 9–14 months. The horse has to be reintroduced to work gradually. Other treatments include injections into the ligaments, pin firing and shock wave treatment.

Related conditions Tendon and ligament strains.

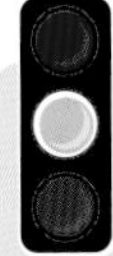

URGENCY INDICATOR

Fairly urgent. Requires early diagnosis.

COST

Depends on the degree of damage. The greater the damage, the higher costs are likely to be.

Lymphangitis

This is a condition that causes swelling of the legs due to restricted lymphatic flow.

Symptoms Very swollen limbs, often associated with lameness.

Causes Reaction to infection, trauma, damage to the tissues post bandaging problems and immobility.

Owner action Veterinary treatment should be sought early on. Bandaging the legs carefully with cold hosing may help in the early stages.

Treatment Cold hosing and pressure bandaging may be useful in the early stages. In some cases, temporary improvement may be seen following exercise and some cases recover spontaneously with rest. Anti-inflammatory drugs and corticosteroids can be useful, and giving antibiotics as a back up is usually advised.

VET CLINIC

Diagnosis is usually made on the basis of visible symptoms, although ultrasound scanning can be helpful in doubtful cases. Most horses will not show severe lameness, although they often resent palpation of the swollen area. There is usually no temperature rise and it is often difficult or impossible to establish the cause.

Related conditions Injuries of the tendon sheath, septic arthritis and cellulites.

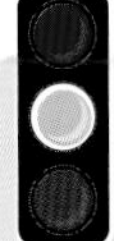

URGENCY INDICATOR

Lymphangitis can be a frustrating condition to treat and early advice should be sought.

COST

Usually low.

Setfast

Setfast, which is also known as azoturia, equine rhabdomyolyis or 'Monday morning disease', has been used to cover a number of conditions. It primarily describes a stiffness of the muscles and can occur in horses of any breed and age.

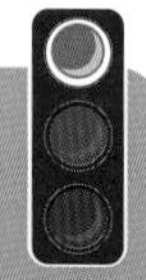

URGENCY INDICATOR

Urgent. This is an acute condition, which must be treated in the early stages. Untreated, it sometimes leads to death of the horse.

COST

Not too expensive as response to treatment is fairly rapid.

Symptoms Stiffness, varying from very mild to extreme, unwillingness to move, collapse.

Causes Exercise is one of the most common trigger factors, but it can be set off by light exercise. Setfast can often be seen in the exhausted horse syndrome, which result from loss of fluids and electrolytes.

Owner action As soon as you notice an unwillingness to perform or walk or any stiffness and cramping, do not force the horse to move. Warm him up with blankets to prevent chilling and seek urgent veterinary assistance.

Treatment Immediate rest. If your horse is a long way from the stable or trailer, he should be transported by horse ambulance or trailer. Forced exercise and prolonged transportation must also be avoided. Initial treatment involves maintaining the fluid balance, possibly using intravenous anti-inflammatories and non-steroidal anti-inflammatories (NSAIDs) to reduce pain.

Small doses of sedation may be necessary to reduce distress, and careful use of muscle relaxants may prove helpful. Careful nursing is necessary to keep the horse warm and dry, and ideally he should not be moved until he has been moving freely around the stable for 24 hours free from symptoms. The horse should not be exercised before the blood analysis of muscle enzymes (see pages 66–67) has improved considerably.

DIAGNOSIS

Diagnosis is made from a history of previous episodes, symptoms of stiffness in movement, tight muscles and pain, and distress on movement. Typically both hindlegs are involved, but occasionally it may be only one hindleg. Early symptoms may be slight, such as slowing down at the end of a race, jumping badly at the end of cross-country or reduced length of stride. Heart rate is elevated. Blood tests are helpful, and even early on they can reveal rises in muscle enzymes. In more extreme cases, coloured urine is passed.

Related conditions Exhausted horse syndrome, muscle strains and sprains.

Prevention Always warm horses up and down before and after competition. Extra care when exercising is needed for horses that have had this problem before. It may be helpful to have the blood monitored regularly for muscle enzymes. During recuperation, reduce the level of high-energy feed appropriate to the amount of work the horse is doing. There is no guaranteed way to prevent horses from suffering from episodes of setfast, but careful management and diet can allow them to continue competing.

Problems of the upper forelimb

Some of the more commonly occurring lamenesses created by the areas of the shoulder, elbow and knee are described below.

Causes Most instances of lameness of the forelimb are caused by lower limb problems. The small number of upper limb lamenesses are caused by trauma.

Owner action Seek veterinary advice at an early stage.

KNEE

The most common type of injury to the knee is caused by trauma, because the knee is not well protected and a falling horse commonly lands on the knees.

The bones of the knee are exposed. The knee is made up of complex rows of bones, which are easily fractured by over-extension of the joint or in a fall. The joint also suffers from degenerative joint disease (see page 75), and occasionally the accessory carpal (the small bone at the back of the knee) is fractured and causes a variable degree of lameness. Swellings found in various areas surrounding the knee are usually the result of trauma and should be treated promptly.

Treatment Wounds to joints should always be treated extremely seriously (see page 75).

ELBOW

The elbow joint is a hinge joint and is a less common source of lameness than the lower joints of the limb. Occasionally capped elbows are seen in horses that have been recumbent for a long time, lying on a floor with poor bedding or sometimes from trauma. It is always wise to check that there is no associated fracture or infection. The point of the elbow can be fractured, particularly in traffic accidents or from kicks, and this produces a very severe lameness.

Treatment Veterinary treatment of these conditions is always necessary.

DIAGNOSIS

This is through lameness investigation techniques (see pages 70–71).

SHOULDER

Conditions of the shoulder are extremely rare and are usually caused by accidents. The most common injury seen is trauma to the point of the shoulder, which causes pain in the function of the shoulder and an unwillingness to move the leg forward. Fractures can also occur but are very rare.

Treatment Any swelling or lameness of the upper forelimb joint should be investigated at an early stage.

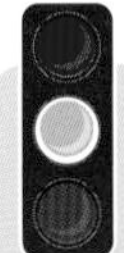

URGENCY INDICATOR

Fairly urgent if the horse is lame.

COST

Cost depends on the cause. It can be fairly high as these problems are often hard to diagnose.

Problems of the upper hindlimb

The conditions described here are among the more commonly occurring types of lameness and trauma of the upper hindlimb joints.

LAMENESS IN THE HOCK

The hock is one of the most common sites of lameness in the hindlimb. The hock is a complicated joint with many large and small bones, of which only one, the hock joint proper, has any significant range of movement. This joint provides the mobility in the hock. The other bones are bound together by strong ligaments but play no part in the bending of the hock. The hock joint proper is a sliding hinge joint.

DIAGNOSIS

Lameness in the hock can be caused by a number of different conditions, and investigations are complex because of the complicated structure of the joint. Lameness of the hock joint proper (the upper mobile part of the joint) is less common than lameness caused by the non-mobile lower areas. The lameness needs to be investigated (see pages 70–71) and joint blocks are useful, before imaging techniques such as X-rays and scans.

BONE SPAVIN

Bone spavin lameness is caused by compression of the specialized bones that make up the lower areas of the hock joint and articulate with the cannon bone. Spavin is due to pathological changes in the cartilage and underlying bony tissue of the small bone plates, and pain occurs when bones are compressed. It is essentially an osteoarthritic condition, and poor conformation has been suggested as an important factor.

Athletic pursuits, such as jumping, obviously put considerable strain on this joint. The onset is often gradual, and symptoms are lameness with, in many cases, no obvious changes on palpation of the area. In severe cases it is possible to feel bony lumps and a change in the seat of spavin on the inside of the hock.

DIAGNOSIS

Bone spavin is confirmed by the use of local anaesthetic injections and X-rays. A 60-second flexion test of the hindlimb will often produce pronounced lameness.

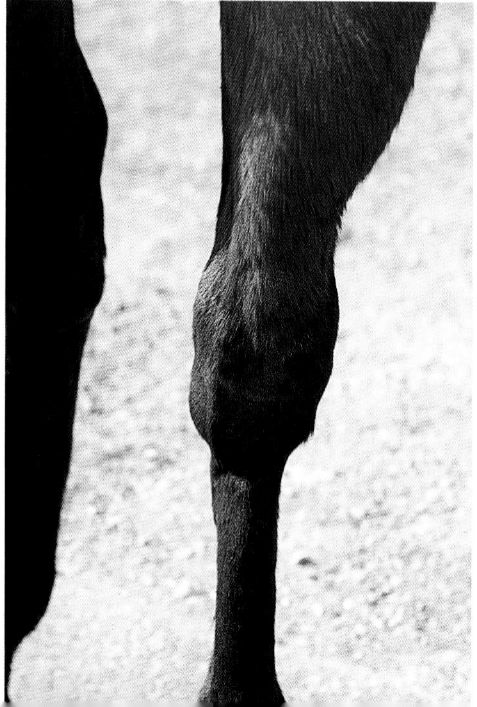

This horse has a bog spavin, the higher of the two bumps on his hock, and a bone spavin, the lower bump.

Treatment This varies according to the condition and its severity. Use of localized injections of non-steroidal and steroidal preparations, as described in the treatment of degenerative joint disease (see page 75), are effective in combination with remedial (surgical) shoeing. In some cases, the area may fuse, and there are surgical techniques that can be used to speed up the fusing process. Once fusion of the joint has occurred lameness often disappears.

BOG SPAVIN

This is a soft swelling of the hock due to distension of the mobile hock joint. It is often seen in hardworking horses with no lameness. It may occur in cases of osteochondritis dessicans (OCD), which requires X-rays or scans to diagnose. Occasionally, bog spavin is seen as a symptom of traumatic injury of the hock joint associated with the tearing of the capsule and, possibly, injury to the joint surface. In these cases lameness is usually evident. If your horse has a large bog spavin, particularly if it suddenly developed on one leg, you should seek veterinary advice.

Treatment Severe OCD and traumatic injury to the joint may require orthopaedic surgery.

CURB

This term is used to describe a swelling on the back of the hock joint below the point of the hock. It is caused by damage to the fibres of the ligament that runs across the back of the hock. Mild lameness is usually noted at the time of the strain but usually settles down quickly and, providing the horse's conformation is good and he does not suffer from sickle or cow hocks, the potential for full recovery is good.

Treatment Rest and local treatment, plus a sensible programme of rehabilitation.

LAMENESS IN THE STIFLE JOINT

The stifle joint corresponds to the human knee. It has two separate articulations and has the kneecap (patella) at the front. The most common source of lameness in the stifle involves the kneecap, which, particularly in horses with poor conformation, can fix in an upward position and prevent the joint from unlocking. The horse then drags his leg and cannot bend it. In severe, recurrent cases, surgery can assist this condition.

The kneecap can also subluxate (move sideways out of the groove and away from the body). This is most common in horses with very straight stifles and is often seen in those that are not physically fit. OCD in the hock is quite common in some breeds, particularly European warmbloods, and sometimes has to be treated surgically. Sometimes the kneecap is hurt in a fall, and this may lead to fracture.

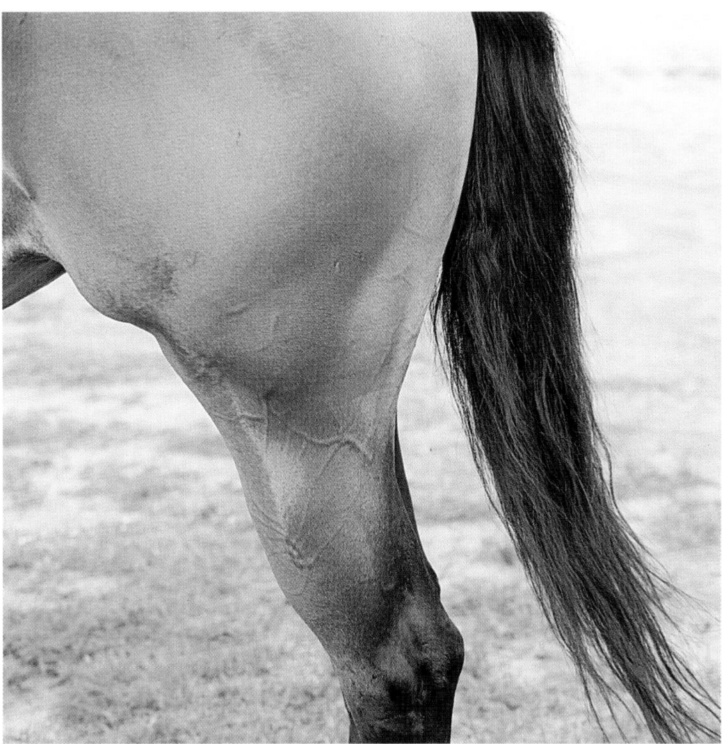

A distension of the stifle area due to joint injury.

Treatment This usually involves careful shoeing and a fitness regime of mainly straight-line work, which does not involve too many tight circles and corners.

LAMENESS IN THE HIP JOINT

This is an unusual site of lameness in the horse because it is protected by a large muscle mass. It occasionally suffers from degenerative joint disease (see page 75) and is sometimes involved in severe pelvic fractures.

Treatment Rest, and possibly anti-inflammatory injections. Physiotheraphy may help.

Stringhalt

This is the sudden snatching up of one or both hindlegs when moving. It is normally more obvious when the horse is walking.

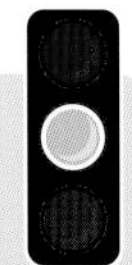

URGENCY INDICATOR

Fairly urgent to rule out any other problems.

 **COST**

Low, as treatment is normally not necessary.

Symptoms Excessive flexion of the hindlimb or limbs, which often occurs every stride. It can be so exaggerated that the horse strikes his stomach. The foot is then held momentarily and then brought sharply downwards.

Causes Stringhalt can develop at any age and its cause in individual animals is unknown. In mild cases the horse may be able to continue work but, although there is no lameness, it is very ungainly. The condition may get progressively worse.

Owner action Seek confirmation of the condition and advice on the degree of severity from your veterinary surgeon.

 **DIAGNOSIS**

The distinctive action is usually enough to diagnose this condition.

Treatment Not usually necessary, but in severe cases surgery can be performed although it is often not particularly satisfactory.

Related conditions Fibrous ossifying myopathy (see below) and shivering.

Note: Australian stringhalt, which has similar symptoms, is believed to be caused by toxic plants and funguses. These cases often recover without treatment.

Fibrous ossifying myopathy

This is relatively rare in the UK, but is more common in the USA in western performance and rodeo horses. It is believed to be related to sliding stops and changes in direction. Similar traumatic injury can occur in road or jumping accidents.

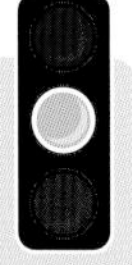

URGENCY INDICATOR

Fairly urgent.

 **COST**

Low if surgery is not required.

Symptoms The characteristic gait is rather like a goose step of marching troops: the hindleg comes forward normally but a split second before it is due to be placed on the ground, it snatches back from a height of 10–20cm (4–8in). It may affect one or both legs and can be difficult to spot.

Causes Tearing of muscle fibres in the hindlimbs, commonly occurring after sharp stops and changes of direction, which puts pressure on the hindleg muscles.

Owner action Ask your veterinary surgeon to check the abnormal gait to confirm diagnosis.

 **DIAGNOSIS**

Examination of the muscle may show evidence of thickened scarring, but in many cases it is difficult to find and the diagnosis can be made on the characteristic stride.

Treatment Several surgical techniques have been used to help severe cases, but they are relatively complicated and the results are somewhat unpredictable.

Related conditions Stringhalt (see above).

Splints

The splint bone is the small bone that extends down either side of the cannon bone at the back of the leg. It articulates at the knee and is held to the cannon bone by a fibrous interosseous ligament. A true splint forms when this ligament is torn, as when it then heals a bony lump forms.

Symptoms Lameness, and a painful hot swelling over the area of injury on the splint bone. Unfortunately, any lump on the splint bone tends to be regarded as a splint, and consequently many fractures and other causes are misdiagnosed.

Causes Splints are caused when the fibrous ligament between the splint bone and the cannon bone is torn. The body mends these types of tears by producing a small, bony lump, which fuses the two bones together. Splints are likely to be caused by conformation and action that put excessive stress on the inside or outside splint bone.

Serious injury sometimes leads to a fracture of the splint bone. This will heal well if there is little displacement, but surgical removal of the bone fragments is sometimes necessary.

Owner action Seek veterinary advice if you notice heat or swelling in the area of the splint and do not work your horse. Mild lameness on a circle is a common symptom.

Treatment Complete box rest for four to six weeks. Topical preparations, such as dimethyl sulphoxide (DMSO) or other anti-inflammatories, can help in the early stages, and careful bandaging is also beneficial. A working blister may help in a later stage. The condition has a good prognosis for recovery.

Related conditions Tendon and ligament conditions affecting the areas below the knee.

COLD SPLINTS

Chronic bony swellings or cold splints are a blemish but do not usually cause lameness. They occasionally put pressure on important surrounding tissues, such as the suspensory ligament, and they can be removed by surgery if necessary.

It is essential that shoes are properly fitted and feet well-balanced, especially in young horses. Tired and unfit young horses should not be overworked on unsuitable surfaces. Apart from surgical treatment, costs are low.

DIAGNOSIS

Examination will reveal a hot, painful swelling in the splint area associated with lameness, which is often more pronounced on hard ground or when the horse is lunged in a circle. Injection of local anaesthetic into the area will confirm the diagnosis, but this is not usually necessary.

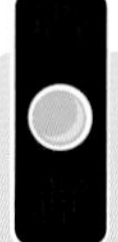

URGENCY INDICATOR

Fairly urgent. Early treatment will reduce the residual bony lump that remains when the splint heals. The sooner the horse is rested, the sooner it will heal and the better the chance of a satisfactory outcome.

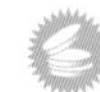

COST

Normally low, unless fractures are involved as these may require surgery.

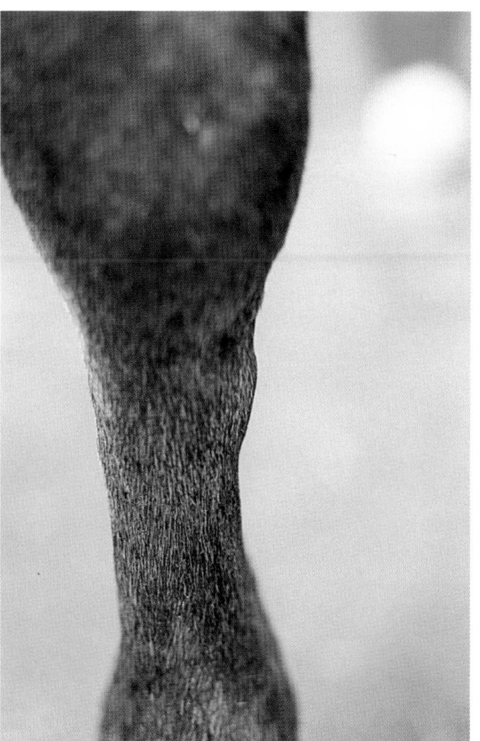

This bony swelling/splint on the side of the cannon bone will cause pain and lameness, and can only be treated with complete box rest.

Back problems

Cases of back pain are always complicated and can arise from a number of other problems that affect the muscles in the back. Hind limb lameness (see pages 80–81) is a common primary factor in back problems.

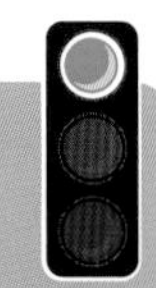

URGENCY INDICATOR

Urgent if the horse is lame or very sore.

COST

Cost depends on the severity of the injury. Mild problems are fairly inexpensive to remedy, whereas chronic conditions can become more expensive.

Symptoms Horses with 'bad back' syndrome are usually reported to have lost performance, often involving a change in action in both ground work and jumping, and sometimes including not making a good shape in the air, cat jumping or dropping a leg while jumping.

Causes Several conditions can produce back pain in the horse and it is often a complex issue, involving other parts of the body. For example, if a horse has sore feet and will not land or jump properly, the change in his action will put more pressure through the shoulders, withers and back and will begin to cause pain in and around the wither area. Similarly, a hock problem, such as spavin, will invariably cause the horse to jump more off one leg than the other, thus twisting the pelvis and putting pressure through the sacroiliac junction between the pelvis and the spine. This can easily result in back pain.

Owner action If you notice that your horse has changed in the way he jumps and moves seek veterinary advice.

Treatment This will depend on the area in which the pain occurs and may involve physiotherapy and manipulation or an injection into localized areas, anti-inflammatory drugs given orally, heat or laser therapy, ultrasound, magnetic therapy and massage. In addition, always make sure that the horse's workload is adjusted to the problem.

Pain relief will allow the horse to move more normally, because much back pain is created through compensation by other muscle masses. The use of gel pads in the area of the saddle may help. Checking that the saddle fits properly and making sure that it is adequately padded is also extremely important.

Related conditions Setfast (see page 78) and traumatic muscle damage.

DIAGNOSIS

Observation of the horse in action should reveal any changes, particularly when he is jumping or performing complicated dressage movements. Pain will often be elicited by careful palpation, but this can be difficult to identify as touching areas of the spine also stimulates normal reflexes. The use of local anaesthesia and local anti-inflammatories may improve the lameness and confirm the diagnosis.

Bone scanning (scintigraphy) and radiography may also be useful, particularly for diagnosing damaged areas of bone and possible fractures of the horse's back after a fall or a severe injury. Ultrasonic diagnosis helps with problems involving the ligaments of the spine.

SPINAL PROBLEMS

Back problems which are directly related to the spine require specific treatment. They include the following:

- **Kissing spines** is a condition where the dorsal spines of the vertebrae rub together as the back flexes, causing inflammation and new bone growth. In some horses this can lead to a reluctance to jump and erratic behaviour. Surgical treatment is occasionally performed for this condition, but it is usually controlled by local injections of anti-inflammatories and physiotherapy.
- **Sacroiliac joint injuries** involve the sacroiliac, a joint with very little movement between the pelvis and the spine. The sacroiliac tends to be torn when the horse exerts a lot of pressure through one hindleg by slipping during jumping or in a fall. The ligaments are torn, which causes pain at the top of the pelvis and produces a change in the action of the hindleg as well as possible lameness.

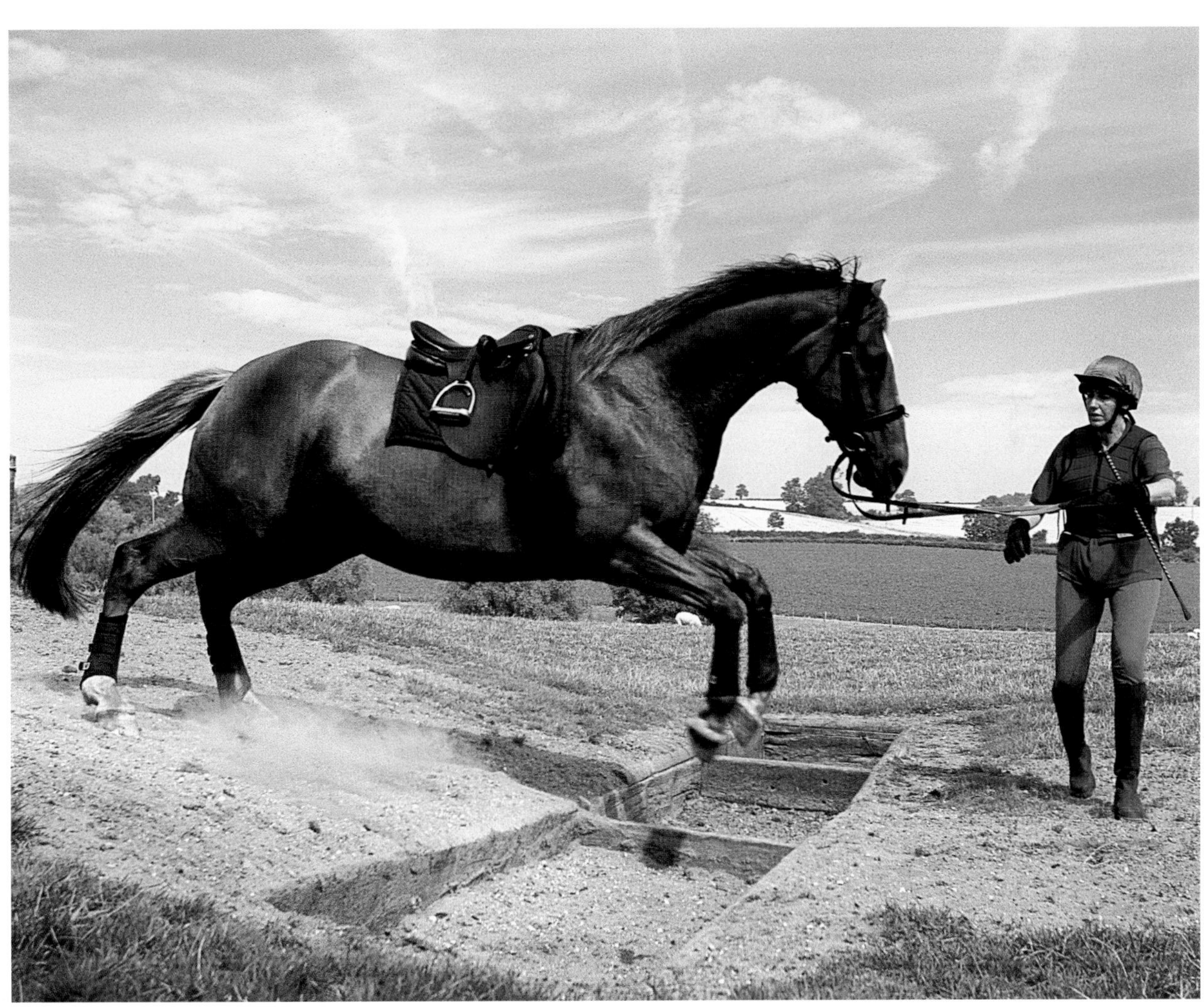

Sacroiliac joint injuries usually respond to deep cortico-steroidal injections, rest and straight-line work during recuperation. Occasionally, recurrent cases require more severe and invasive treatment. This is a common problem in the competition horse.

Observing the horse while jumping will show his back extension and help to reveal any back problems.

Neck injuries

Neck trauma is usually the result of a fall while jumping and is most severe when the horse falls with a flexed neck. There may be instantaneous damage to the spinal cord causing paralysis, ataxia and death, or more minor injuries causing neck pain.

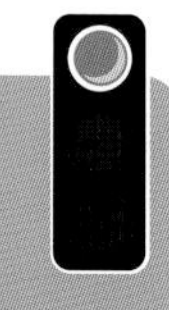

URGENCY INDICATOR

Very urgent.

COST

Depends on the degree of damage and whether surgical intervention is required.

Symptoms Unable to stand, or if able to stand the horse cannot move his neck. May be very uncoordinated or even paralysed.

Causes Normally caused by a traumatic injury, for example a fall. Neck injuries in a foal may be caused by being trodden on.

Owner action If the horse is at all wobbly when walking in a straight line, even if this is mild, seek immediate veterinary advice.

Treatment If there is marked staggering and an inability to walk, urgent veterinary treatment is required and the horse's future is determined by the speed at which he improves in response to treatment.

Horses that have severe tearing and bruising of the muscles can be difficult to diagnose accurately at the time of the fall, and so are normally rested and treated with anti-inflammatory medication. This is not always advisable because movement during healing is unwise. If a fracture is suspected, the horse would normally be fed at head level to prevent movement. The future for horses with fractures of the neck depends on the location of the injury and what other areas are involved. Physiotherapy and a good mobilization plan to keep the muscles moving and prevent stiffness are important for muscular injuries of the neck.

DIAGNOSIS

This can be extremely complicated, particularly if the horse is unable to lift his head and neck after a fall. There may be absence of nerve reflexes, which may have been caused by damage to the nerves affected by the fall. If the horse is standing, the tilt of the head and neck may indicate painful areas that have been damaged during the fall and should be carefully examined. It is important to check whether the horse is stable on his feet and is able to balance.

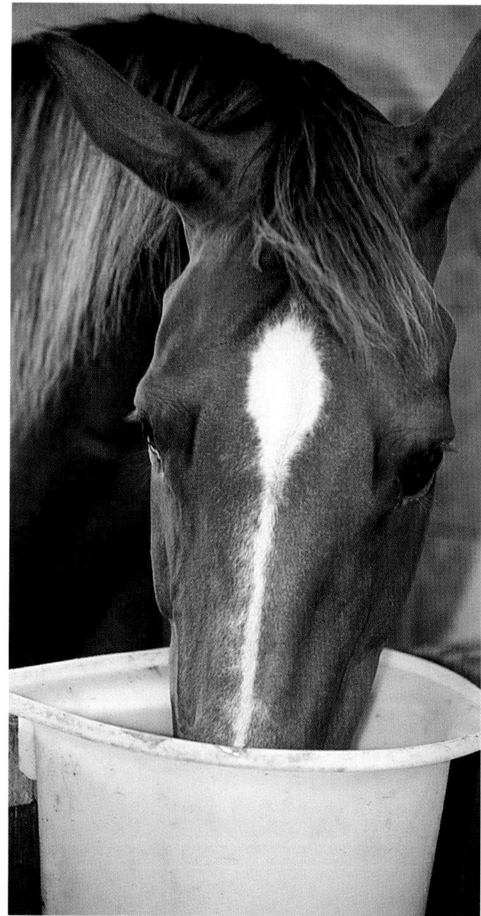

Feed the horse at head level in order to minimize any movement of the neck.

Head injuries

Some of the traumatic injuries to the head have been discussed in the sections of this book dealing with the eye and the mouth.

Symptoms Wounds, swellings, haemorrhage from the wounds or nose and concussion. There may be other neurological symptoms, such as loss of balance. Some of the symptoms may be of delayed onset.

Causes This type of injury is usually caused by falls during jumping or road traffic accidents.

Owner action All head injuries are serious and should receive veterinary attention. Observe any changes in mental state or behaviour and always treat horses that have had a head injury with great care because they may respond violently. Always make sure the airway is clear.

Treatment This will depend on the results of the clinical and neurological examinations (see page 88). First aid treatment should be given for any wound or bleeding and anti-inflammatories and cortico-steroids may be used to reduce inflammation that may cause pressure on other vital organs in the head. Sedation may also be required if the horse suffers from behavioural changes. A suspected fracture of the skull should be referred for radiology and possible surgical repair. Most fractures of the jaw respond well to surgery.

DIAGNOSIS

Diagnosis depends on observation of the injuries. It is important to have veterinary assistance and this will often include a neurological examination.

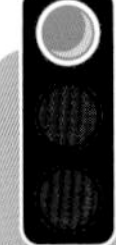

URGENCY INDICATOR

Very urgent.

COST

Depends on the degree of secondary investigation required and possible surgical procedures.

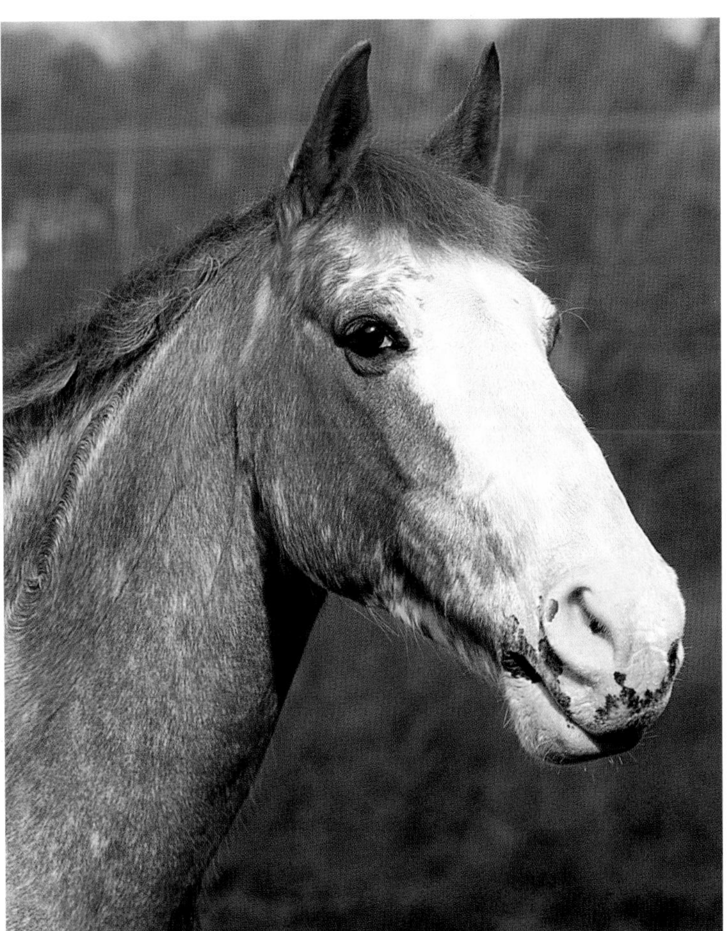

All injuries to the horse's head should be regarded as serious and receive veterinary attention as quickly as possible.

The nervous system

To understand neurological problems it is necessary to know a little about the basic nervous system of the horse. If some sort of stimulus is applied to the surface of the body, a message is carried by the local peripheral nerves to the spinal cord and then to the brain stem, where it is analysed in the appropriate area of the brain. The brain then reacts by relaying the information back down the spinal cord to the peripheral nerves, and then to the muscles, instructing them how to move.

Neurological conditions are caused by damage to or pressure on the nerve tracks, and examination involves taking a careful case history and carrying out a physical examination to assess the horse's demeanour, responsiveness, head position and ability to turn and back, both with and without a blindfold. Limb weakness, particularly hind-end weakness, and the ability to walk up and down slopes will also be assessed. The inclination of the head when walking up and down slopes can show if there is any spasticity (stiffness).

The domesticated horse retains many of the instincts of his wild forebears, and fear and flight are two of the strongest of these. Many behavioural problems are created by the environment and regimes to which modern working horses are exposed. In the wild the horse is a herd animal, and isolation and boredom are contributory factors in a number of equine vices, including weaving, crib biting and wind sucking. A good living and working environment will prevent many of these traits from developing.

Weaving occurs when a bored horse develops the habit of moving his head from side to side in the stable doorway. A door grill may help to prevent this, but horses often continue to weave inside the stable. The habit can be picked up by other horses in the yard.

Some horses hold on to mangers or the door, which is known as crib biting, and suck air. This latter habit often develops into wind sucking, which is when the horse no longer needs to hold on to an object to suck air. Both conditions are brought on by boredom and often cause loss of condition, abnormal wear of the teeth and colic.

So that your horse is never bored you must provide small, frequent meals, toys to play with and regular attention.

Quick-reference guide to ailments in this chapter:

Wobbler's syndrome

This is an inability to co-ordinate limb action, particularly hindlimb action, because of pressure from the abnormal growth of the bones in the neck.

Symptoms This condition is usually seen in younger horses, and mostly affects thoroughbreds and quarter horses, although warmbloods may also exhibit this problem. Wobbler's syndrome is more frequent in males than females and is often found in horses that are well grown for their age.

There is often a history of poor performance, stumbling or falling, and ataxia (difficulty standing) and weakness are the predominant symptoms. These symptoms are most noticeable when the horse is walking up or down slopes or in a circle. If the tail is pulled while the horse is walking, the hindquarters tend to sway.

Radiographs will quite often show up some bony abnormality in the cervical vertical column. Confirmation is through demonstrating a reduction in the width of the spinal cord by injecting a dye into the spinal cord, which will highlight its exact dimensions.

Causes Compression of the spinal cord and nerve tracks by an abnormal bone growth in the neck. There have been many suggested causes, including genetics, mineral imbalance and nutrition.

DIAGNOSIS

Diagnosis is based on clinical symptoms and radiographic findings.

Owner action If you have a young horse that is unsteady in his action, seek veterinary advice.

Treatment Medical management to stabilize the condition with the use of painkillers and anti-inflammatories may be useful if the onset is sudden. Some horses respond to prolonged rest, but the condition is often progressive. Surgical procedures have been attempted but with only a moderate degree of success so far.

Related conditions Neck injuries (see page 86), equine herpes (see page 90), neuritis, rabies (see page 94) and worm damage to the spinal cord.

WARNING Wobbler's syndrome can be dangerous because horses affected by it can fall unexpectedly.

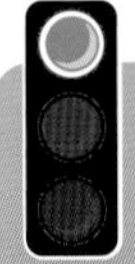

URGENCY INDICATOR

Urgent.

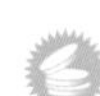

COST

Often expensive, especially if surgery is needed.

Equine herpes

This virus has four subtypes causing differing symptoms. EHV1 causes respiratory symptoms, abortions, ataxia and possible paralysis. EHV2 can cause mild respiratory symptoms and poor performance. EHV3 causes coital exanthema, and EHV4 causes respiratory disease.

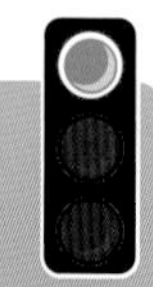

URGENCY INDICATOR

Urgent.

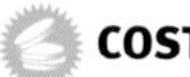

COST

May be expensive due to prolonged treatment.

Symptoms Weakness, wobbliness and, in some cases, collapse. The horse may not be able to pass urine properly.

Causes Myeloencephalopathy is an equine herpes virus that causes an inflammation of the vessels in the central nervous system.

Owner action Urgent veterinary attention is needed. Because this virus is so infectious, isolate your horse.

Treatment It is critical that the horse receives supportive therapy. Horses that have collapsed are difficult to treat and have the worst chance of recovery. Horses with urinary retention require both catheterization and intensive nursing, and recovery may take many weeks. Some horses' symptoms persist after recovery.

Related conditions Neuritis, wobbler's syndrome (see page 89), meningitis, trauma, rabies (see page 94), congenital abnormalities and brain abcesses.

DIAGNOSIS

There will be a history of exposure to respiratory virus or abortion. It may appear in a single horse or occur in an outbreak. Respiratory infection usually occurs 10–14 days before the onset of weakness. Blood tests will prove positive to the virus.

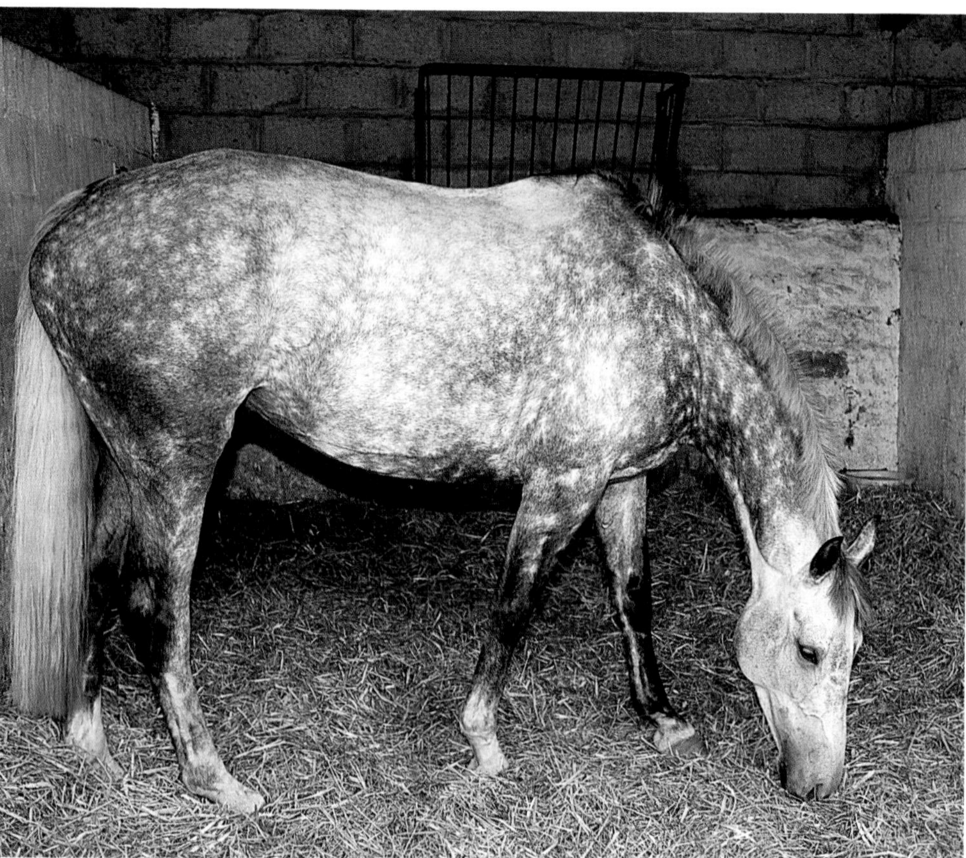

Isolate your horse immediately in order to prevent the extremely infectious herpes virus from spreading.

Head shaking

Except in the most severe cases, head shaking becomes a clinical problem only when the horse is being ridden. It may be instinctive or part of normal sexual or avoidance behaviour.

Symptoms Nodding of the head or head shaking by the horse at rest or in exercise.

Causes Any problem that causes irritation or pain in the head area may cause this type of behaviour. Specific causes are discovered in only a few cases. These typically include space-occupying growths, like tumours, inflammatory or degenerative conditions in the sinuses, guttural pouch or nose and mouth areas, and inflammation of the nerve tracks to the head areas, particularly to the face and teeth.

Owner action Seek veterinary advice if there is abnormal head nodding or shaking that cannot be put down to resistance to the training processes or environment.

DIAGNOSIS

This is made on the symptoms exhibited and the cause is treated appropriately.

Treatment Because of the complicated nature of this condition, it is important to perform an extensive examination to rule out the problems listed above. If those problems are identified as a cause, then they can be treated on an individual basis.

Related conditions Fly problems, ear mites and behavioural problems.

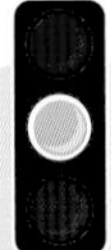

URGENCY INDICATOR

Fairly urgent. The degree of urgency depends on the symptoms and the underlying cause, but the earlier that causes are identified the better.

COST

Expensive because of the extensive nature of the necessary examinations.

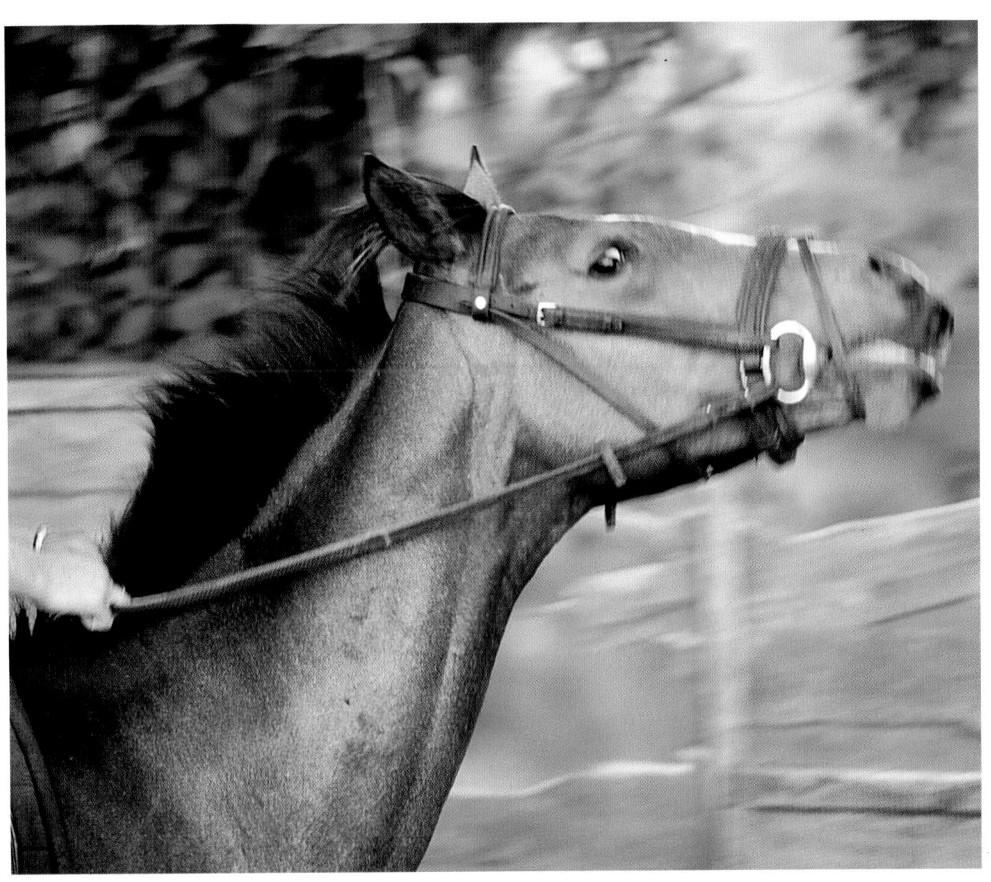

There are numerous possible causes for head shaking, which can be distressing for both horse and rider.

Equine degenerative myeloencephalopathy (EDM)

In some parts of the world this condition has been found to be evident in more than 20 per cent of horses examined at post mortem that have had a history of ataxia (difficulty standing). It is most likely to be seen in foals born to dams that have previously had foals with this condition.

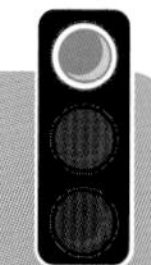

URGENCY INDICATOR

Urgent, due to the distress the horse will suffer.

 **COST**

Cost of euthanasia will be required.

Symptoms The symptoms of ataxia and paralysis are variable but are usually noticeable before the horse is 12 months old. All limbs are commonly affected, although it is usually worse in the hindlimbs.

Causes Not completely known, but a number of factors have been implicated such as dirty yards, insecticides, wood preservatives and lack of vitamin E.

Owner action These symptoms require immediate veterinary attention.

 **DIAGNOSIS**

A clinical diagnosis will be necessary.

Treatment Once signs have developed, this condition is extremely difficult to treat. Providing a good diet that is high in vitamin E may be useful, as lack of vitamin E has been implicated as a causal factor.

Equine protozoa myeloencephalopathy (EPM)

This is a debilitating and potentially fatal disease caused by a protozoa. It is most commonly seen in horses younger than four years, but can be seen in all ages.

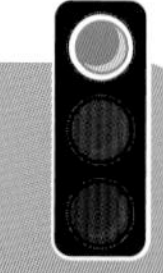

URGENCY INDICATOR

Urgent, due to the distress the horse will suffer.

 **COST**

Expensive, as often a long duration of therapy is needed.

Symptoms Onset of symptoms is usually acute and progressive, with stumbling and frequent falling. It is most common in the midwest, northeast and south of America. This condition is not seen in the UK.

Causes A protozoan (*Sarcocystis neurona*) invades the body's cells, eventually affecting the muscles and cranial nerves.

Owner action These symptoms require immediate veterinary attention.

Treatment Medical treatment can be effective but is often required over a long period of time.

 **DIAGNOSIS**

Diagnosis is extremely difficult. It is done on clinical signs and response to therapy. It is possible to diagnose the condition at post mortem, where lesions are found in the spinal cord and brain.

Tetanus

Also called lockjaw, tetanus is an extremely serious and often fatal disease, which is caused by a bacterium commonly found in the soil (among other places), where the spores may persist for many years. Contaminated wounds and penetrations are the main source of problems.

Symptoms Restricted jaw movements, prolapsed third eyelid and unsteady straddling gait. The tail is often held out stiffly, particularly when moving and turning. An anxious alert expression with dilated nostrils, exaggerated response to stimulation, difficulty in eating and an unwillingness to eat, often with saliva dribbling from the mouth, are characteristic.

Causes The bacterium *Clostridium tetani*, which produces exotoxins and grows rapidly in the environment created by a penetrating wound. The exotoxins enter the nervous system and result in muscular spasticity and exaggerated responses, leading to paralysis of essential functions and death.

Owner action With any cut, no matter how small, veterinary advice should be sought and the horse's tetanus vaccine status checked.

Treatment Treatment aims to eliminate the causative organism, neutralize residual toxins and control the symptoms produced by the effect of the toxin on the nerves. Veterinary treatment will vary according to symptoms, but it is likely to involve the use of antibiotics, anti-toxins, sedatives and painkillers. It is also necessary to keep a close eye on dehydration. Fluids and food may have to be administered either intravenously or by stomach tube. There is always a grave prognosis with tetanus cases.

DIAGNOSIS

Diagnosis is usually made from the characteristic symptoms. Incubation may be one to three weeks, but unfortunately locating the site of infection is extremely difficult.

Related conditions Laminitis (see page 74), setfast (see page 78), hypocalcaemia and heatstroke.

WARNING All horses must be regularly vaccinated against this dreadful disease.

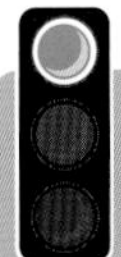

URGENCY INDICATOR

Urgent. Tetanus must be treated immediately if there is to be any hope of the horse recovering.

COST

Potentially very high because of the need for complex support therapy.

Rabies

Rabies is an extremely unpleasant and fatal disease that can affect all warm-blooded domestic species, as well as human beings. It is a virus that attacks the nervous system, with devastating and fatal consequences.

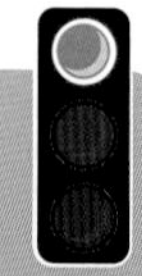

URGENCY INDICATOR

Very urgent. Any symptoms that suggest rabies in areas where the disease is endemic require urgent veterinary advice and attention. In endemic areas vaccination is advisable.

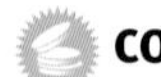

COST

Cost of euthanasia will be required.

Symptoms Symptoms are varied and not specific. They may include tremors and behavioural changes, which may include aggression and self-mutilation. There may be obscure lameness, with wobbly or partly paralysed action. There may be signs of depression, with or without colic, and ultimately death within one to two weeks of onset of symptoms.

Cause The rabies virus ascends the tracts within the nervous system, usually initially producing local hyperactivity (such as tremors) and then at a latter stage causing failure of nerve activity, leading to death. The form the disease takes depends on a number of complicated factors, but it may be seen in a furious form, where the cerebral areas are affected, a dumb form, where the brain stem is affected, or a paralytic form, where the spinal cord is affected.

Owner action If rabies is suspected, great caution must be exercised in handling the horse, because of the risk of disease spread to the handler.

DIAGNOSIS

It is very difficult to identify rabies in a horse because of the lack of specific symptoms. Diagnosis in the live horse is extremely difficult and positive diagnosis depends on laboratory analysis at post mortem.

Treatment There is no successful treatment for rabies at present.

Related conditions Trauma, other viral, parasitic (herpes virus), tetanus or bacterial conditions affecting the nervous system, and hepato encephalopathy.

WARNING Rabies should always be considered in any rapidly progressive neurological disorder in the horse, particularly in areas of the world where it is endemic in the wildlife.

Synchronized diaphragmatic flutter (SDF)

A nervous condition commonly seen in stressed competition horses.

Symptoms A twitch in the flank area, which is synchronized with the heartbeat. This may be accompanied by an audible thump.

Causes Most commonly seen in dehydrated, exhausted horses. The cause is electrolyte deficit or disturbance, which causes nerve irritability that affects the diaphragm and heart. Low calcium levels may also contribute to the nerve irritability.

Owner action Seek immediate veterinary attention if abnormal twitching in the flank or thumps are noticed.

Treatment Correction of the electrolyte imbalances is extremely important, and this is usually performed by giving intravenous fluids, which may include calcium preparations. It is important to monitor the heart during treatment. Fluid therapy alone often restores the intracellular fluid and circulating blood volume, and thereby allows the electrolyte disturbance to self-correct.

DIAGNOSIS

Diagnosis is based on symptoms in horses that have been heavily exercised. A twitch in the flank area is synchronized with the heartbeat, and this may be marked enough to produce an audible thump – hence the common name, thumps. This in itself is not harmful, but it indicates an electrolyte disturbance that must be rapidly corrected because such an imbalance can have fatal consequences.

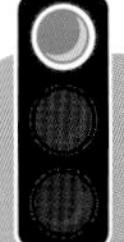

URGENCY INDICATOR

Urgent.

COST

Inexpensive.

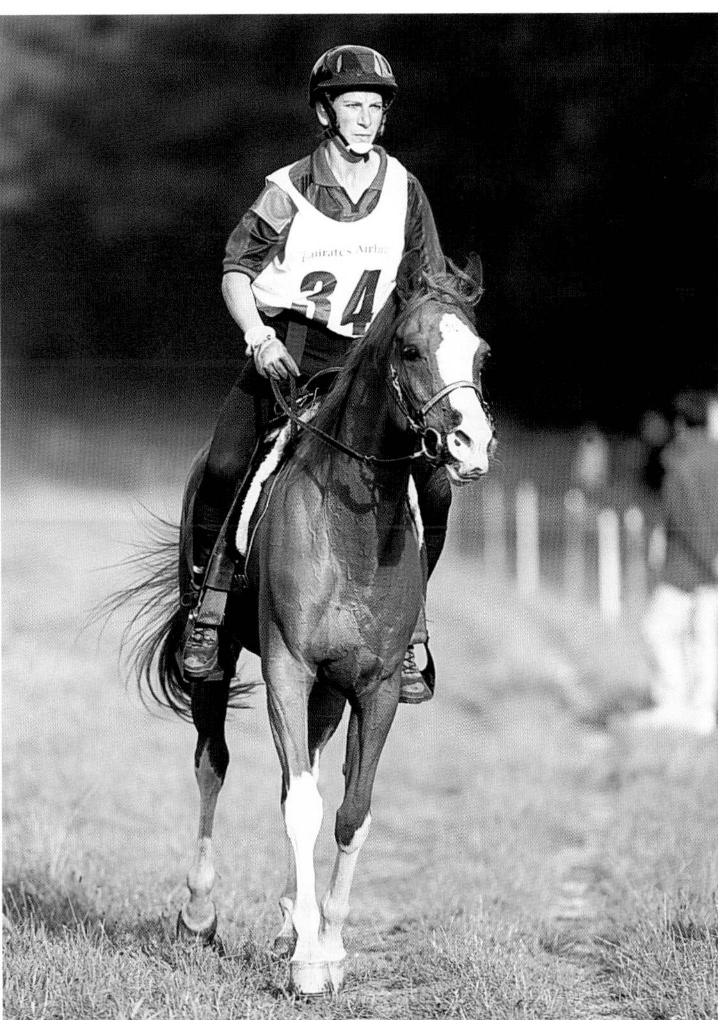

Heavily exercised horses, such as endurance horses, are particularly prone to SDF and keeping them well hydrated is vital.

Travel sickness

Horses that travel long distances by road and air are particularly susceptible to travel sickness, especially if the ventilation and air quality are poor, or if they are unable to put their heads down as they will be unable to clear their airways.

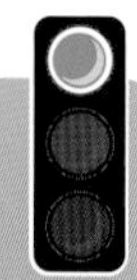

URGENCY INDICATOR

Urgent.

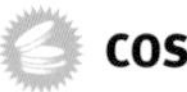

COST

Usually low.

Symptoms The horse will become depressed and stop eating and drinking. This may occur during travel or up to several days afterwards. The horse may run a temperature, have mild, colic-like pains and reduced gut sounds. The pulse will usually be raised by 50 beats per minute or more, and sweating and occasionally an increased respiratory rate will be observed.

Causes Stress is the predisposing factor, particularly when horses that are travelling long distances in crates cannot get their heads down and when the environment, over time, tends to become contaminated and the air quality poor.

Owner action Call for veterinary attention as soon as symptoms are noticed.

Treatment Antibiotics, penicillin sodium, gentamyacin, trimethroprim, steroidalanti-inflammatory drugs, fluids (both intravenously and by stomach tube, possibly with liquid paraffin), and laxative foods are all possibilities. As long as treatment is undertaken early and is accompanied by complete rest and recuperation, the outcome is usually very satisfactory. Pleurisy can be a serious complication.

DIAGNOSIS

Diagnosis is based on the clinical symptoms found in horses that have travelled long distances by road or air.

Related conditions Respiratory infections of other types and colic (see pages 44–45).

Prevention Reduce travel time, where possible, and take proper breaks. Improve the horse's travel environment by using good stalls, and maintain good air quality and a cool temperature throughout the journey. Reducing bulk feed and giving a laxative feed before loading can also help. During the journey, supply small and regular feeds and plenty of fresh water. Premedications before long air or sea trips may also be useful.

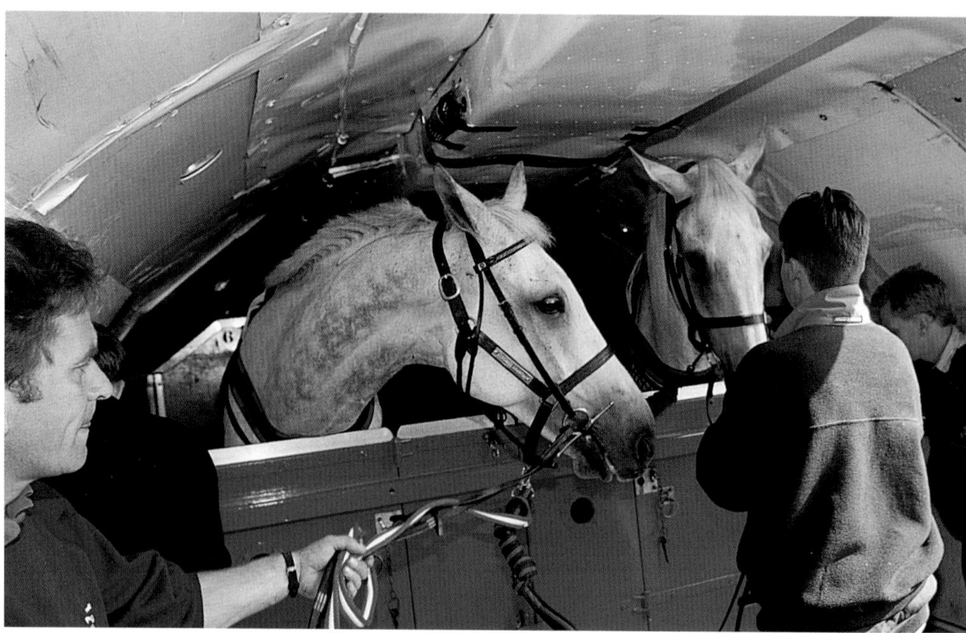

Travelling in an aeroplane can be a stressful experience for a horse, so careful planning is vital.

Transit tetani

Also known as hypocalcaemia, this condition is caused by low calcium and is most frequent in lactating mares or horses in prolonged transport or stressful environments.

Symptoms The severity of the symptoms partly depends on the calcium concentration in the blood and body tissues. Symptoms are stiff gait, profuse sweating, muscle tremors and collapse, weakness of the hindlimbs, unwillingness or difficulty in eating or drinking, salivation, signs of anxiety, increased heart rate, occasionally convulsions and coma that can lead to death.

Cause Low calcium levels.

Owner action Seek immediate veterinary advice if you notice slight changes in character or stiffness, and anxiety in brood or lactating mares and horses that are in transport and are stressed.

DIAGNOSIS

Diagnosis can be backed up by blood tests showing low calcium values. In addition, low magnesium and phosphorus may be seen.

Treatment Veterinary administration of calcium solutions, which may have to be repeated over several days, usually produces good results. Relapses can occur. Mildly affected horses may recover without treatment.

Related conditions Trauma, tetanus (see page 93), hepato encephalopathy and viral, bacterial and parasitic problems affecting the nervous system.

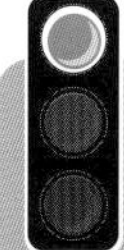

URGENCY INDICATOR

Urgent – transit tetani is life threatening.

COST

Relatively low.

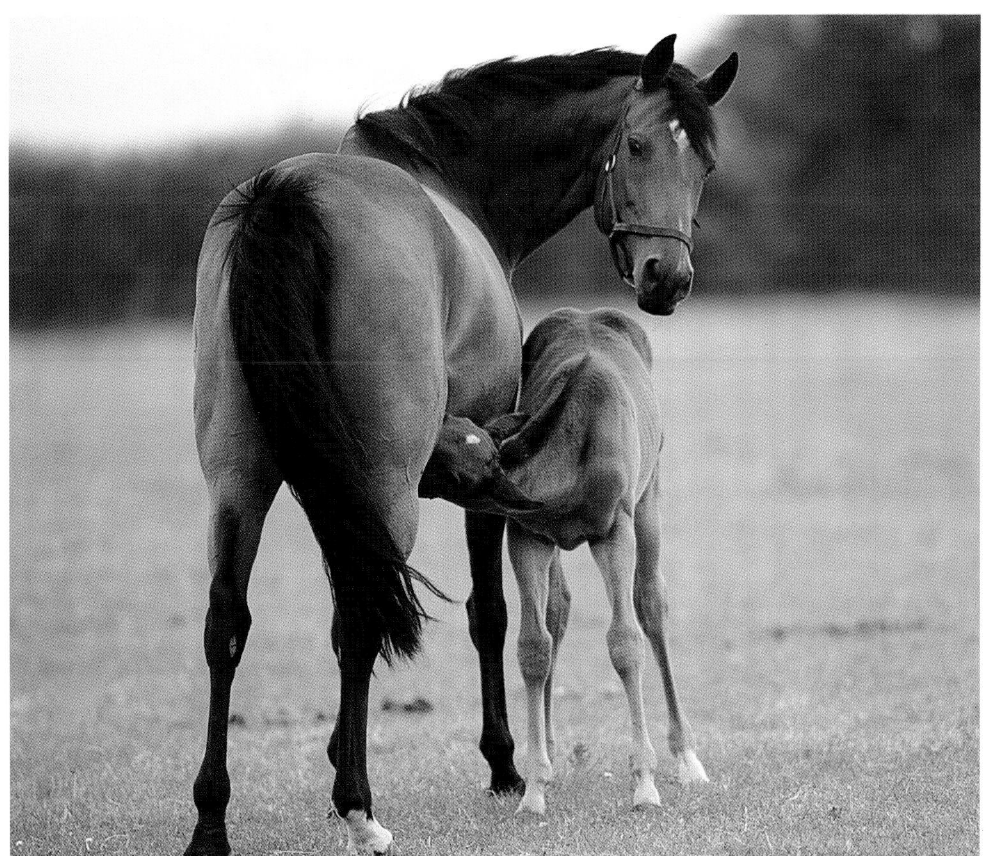

Low calcium levels are most commonly found in mares that are feeding foals.

The male horse

In the male horse, the testicles descend before birth, and it is unlikely that they will drop after birth unless they are sitting very close to the scrotum. The testicles start to increase in size from the age of 12 months, and puberty occurs any time between the ages of 14 months and two years. The horse normally reaches maximum reproductive capacity by the time he is four years old, and after that there is usually no change in the daily sperm production until he is 20 years old.

The penis starts from just below the anus, but the only part that is visible is that which lies within the sheath. This is covered by a piece of skin called the preputial fold. The sheath is very large and often makes a sucking noise when the horse trots.

Debris from the glands and the skin lining the sheath accumulate and form smegma deep within the sheath. The penis and sheath should never be washed in strong antiseptic solutions, which will kill off the normal microbial population living there and predispose the sheath to infections. Use warm water instead.

A cryptorchid, a male horse with one or two undescended testicles, is commonly known as a 'rig'. It is sometimes possible to feel the testicle sitting in the inguinal region, and this is known as an inguinal testicle. Sometimes, however, the testicle is in the abdominal cavity.

Cryptorchids behave like stallions and can be fertile. However, they should be castrated because the testicles in the abdominal cavity will be at a higher temperature than those in the cooler scrotum, and this can induce testicular tumours. There also appears to be a genetic link, which will be passed on if the animal is used for breeding. Cryptorchids can be difficult to handle and are sometimes dangerous.

If a horse with no known history is behaving like a stallion, a blood test will check the hormone levels and show whether the horse has been castrated successfully or whether he is, in fact, a cryptorchid.

Quick-reference guide to ailments in this chapter:

For **swellings**, see pages 99–100

For **castration**, see page 101

Swollen sheath

The sheath of the horse should be checked daily for any change in size, feel or temperature. As the sheath is one of the lowest tissue masses in the body, it tends to become swollen very easily due to the pull of gravity.

Symptoms Swollen sheath and possible heat change or change in consistency.

Causes Infection, tumour of the sheath or penis, trauma, oedema. Also fly or snake bites.

Owner action Try to examine or view the penis to check for lumps. Check for any other swellings on the body.

Treatment This depends on the cause, and may just require antibiotics and washes.

Related conditions Generalized oedema (see page 65) and systemic granulomatous disease.

DIAGNOSIS

Full clinical examination, swabs for bacterial culture and blood tests.

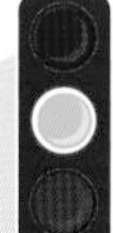

URGENCY INDICATOR

Fairly urgent, or very urgent if the horse is straining to urinate.

COST

Depends on the cause, but normally not too expensive.

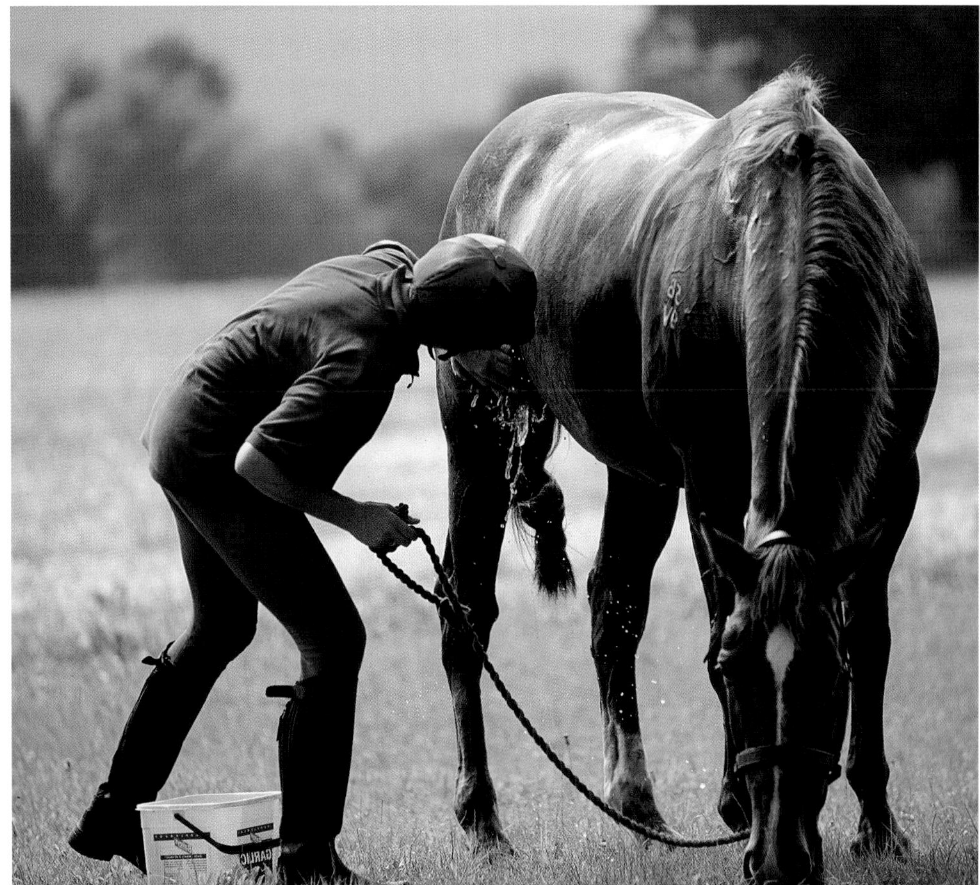

When washing the horse's sheath it is very important to use plain warm water rather than an antiseptic solution.

Testicular swellings

The testicles of entire stallions should be checked every day, and any change in size or position noted.

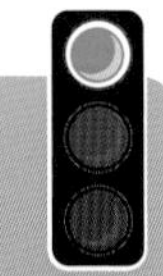

URGENCY INDICATOR

Urgent, especially if associated with colic. Hernias can trap sections of the intestine, which die, requiring immediate surgery.

 **COST**

Depends on the cause. If surgery is required this will be more expensive.

Symptoms Unilateral or bilateral swellings in the testicular region, colic, difficulty urinating.

Causes Hernia, tumours, swelling after trauma, infection, torsion (twisting).

Owner action Seek veterinary advice immediately.

Treatment This depends on the cause. Hernias need urgent surgery, tumours must be removed, and infections require antibiotics and sometimes surgical drainage.

Related conditions Hernia, tumours, swelling after trauma, infection, torsion (twisting).

 **DIAGNOSIS**

Full clinical examination, ultrasound examination of the lump and biopsies may be needed.

Penile paralysis

Due to its anatomical position, the shaft of the penis is easily traumatized. When swollen, the penis may not be able to drop, or if dropped, may not be able to be pulled up. The longer the penis stays out, the more swollen it can get.

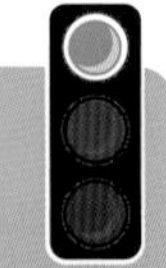

URGENCY INDICATOR

Urgent.

 **COST**

Initial treatment is not expensive, but if there is a slow recovery then nursing costs will be fairly high.

Symptoms Swollen prolapsed penis, colic, difficult urinating.

Causes Trauma, post testicular surgery complication, post-sedation. The shaft of the penis is easily traumatized due to its position, and entire males are very susceptible to being kicked when covering mares.

Owner action Seek immediate veterinary help.

Treatment The penis is covered with an aqueous cream and supported in a sling. Sometimes a urinary catheter may be inserted. Anti-inflammatories, antibiotics and massage are also helpful.

 **DIAGNOSIS**

This is based on clinical signs such as a prolapsed penis, which becomes engorged with blood, is very swollen and sore, and cannot be retracted back into the sheath.

Castration

Castration is the surgical excision of both of the testicles of an entire stallion, and should always be performed by a vet.

Castration is usually carried out when the horse is one to two years old, although it can be done at any age. Castration helps to eliminate some of the masculine characteristics of a stallion, but sometimes these traits are retained, especially in older animals that will already have learned them.

There are two main ways in which to carry out the procedure: in a standing animal using sedation, and in a recumbent animal using general anaesthesia.

Both testicles are removed. Sometimes they are removed still encased in their tunic (a closed castration); alternatively, the tunic may be incised and the testicles removed (an open castration). Whichever method is used, the wound is the same and it is usually left open to drain, although it can be stitched. Different vets carry out different procedures, and there are pros and cons for each method.

A newly castrated male should not be left with mares for six weeks, because he may still have some residual fertile sperm.

Complications

Post-operative swelling: It is normal for a small amount of swelling to appear around the testicle, but this generally recedes within two to three days. It is always worth speaking to the vet if you are worried. If the horse appears ill or if pus is draining from the wound, contact your vet immediately.

Post-operative bleeding: It is fairly common for blood to drip from the wound for up to two hours, but if there is a stream of blood contact your vet as soon as possible.

Tissue hanging from wound: Contact your vet immediately if anything appears from the wound and is hanging down. Because the scrotal sac communicates with the abdomen, the contents of the abdomen sometimes fall though the castration incision. If this happens, make sure the horse is on clean bedding. If a lot of tissue is dangling. try to place some form of body bandage over the horse to hold the tissue to the body, to prevent him from standing on it before the vet arrives.

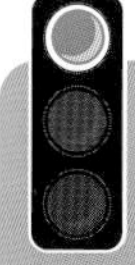

URGENCY INDICATOR

Urgent if there are post-operative complications.

COST

Fairly expensive.

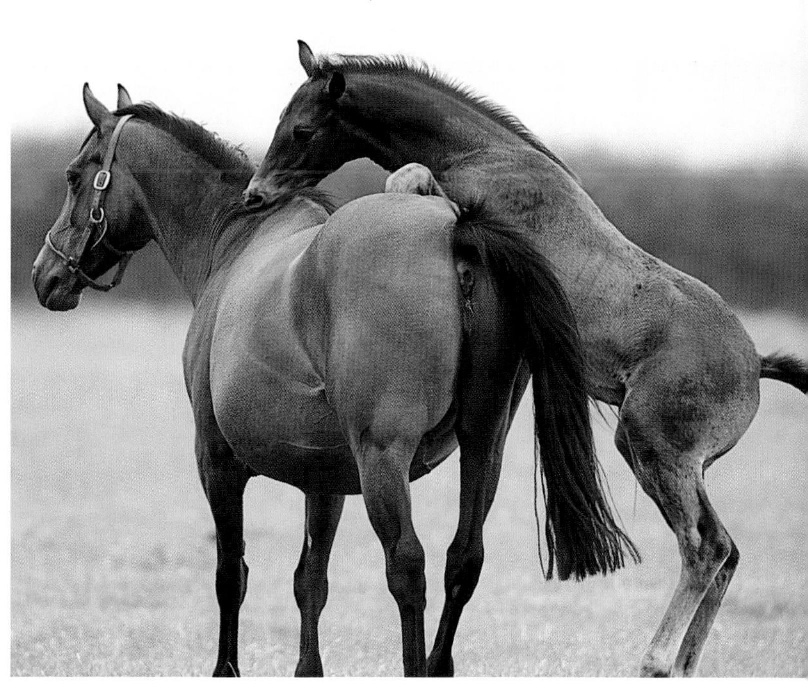

Colts that have not been castrated can be a problem as they may be more frisky or aggressive.

The mare

The mare's reproductive organs are situated within the pelvic and abdominal cavities. Most mares reach sexual maturity when they are two years old, but it can happen earlier. If, for example, a foal is born very early in the year, it is not uncommon for them to have started their cycle by late summer of the following year. However, it is not recommended that young mares are used for breeding purposes because they often do not have a regular cycle until they are three years old.

A normal mare's cycle will occur in late spring, summer and autumn because it is stimulated by the number of hours of daylight. Most mares therefore foal in spring and early summer, and the natural breeding season is from late spring to early summer. Some mares do, however, continue to cycle throughout the winter. In thoroughbred horses the foal's birthday is taken from 1 January, and most thoroughbreds are bred to foal as close to this date as possible.

The average oestrus cycle lasts for 22 days but it is variable, often being longer in spring and shorter in summer. The cycle consists of the follicular phase (also known as oestrus), which lasts for about six days, and the luteal phase (also known as di-oestrus), which lasts for 14–15 days. The mare is receptive to the stallion throughout oestrus: the vulva appears relaxed, the tail is frequently lifted and the clitoris is everted (winking).

Mares can become aggressive and difficult – sometimes impossible – to handle during oestrus. Some mares also have prolonged oestrus. If the mare is not to be used for breeding, it is possible to prolong the di-oestrus with hormones and help to eliminate these behavioural problems.

Quick-reference guide to ailments in this chapter:

For **brood mare and foaling**, see pages 103–106

For **foal problems**, see pages 107–109

The brood mare

In order for a mare to conceive successfully, she needs to be physically healthy, free from sexually transmitted diseases and cycling properly.

Sexually transmitted diseases

Both mare and stallion can carry a number of sexually transmitted diseases, which cause illness in both animals as well as infertility. It is advisable, therefore, to have both tested for these diseases before breeding commences. Testing is compulsory on many stud farms.

Commonly tested diseases

Contagious equine metritis (CEM) CEM causes an infection in the uterus about two days after insemination and leads to the death of the embryo. If it is not treated promptly, infected mares can become carriers and infect the stallion. A clitoral fossa and, sometimes, a uterine swab are taken from the mare, and urethral fossa, urethra, prejaculatory fluid and penile sheath swabs are taken from the stallion.

Equine viral arteritis (EVA) EVA is the most commonly sexually transmitted disease. It causes abortion, accompanied by respiratory problems, conjunctivitis and oedema of the limbs, often occurring at 10–14 days. The disease can also be spread in the air, and a mare infected later in pregnancy may also abort. The disease is tested for by blood tests of the mare and stallion. Breeding stallions can be vaccinated against EVA.

Fertilization

There are three ways a mare can be fertilized. You can allow the mare to run with a stallion, until she becomes pregnant; this is known as pasture breeding. Hand mating is when the stallion is presented to a mare in oestrus. Artificial insemination can also be used, especially among thoroughbreds.

Scanning a mare's ovaries makes it possible to measure the size of the follicles, which will ovulate and produce an egg, and this helps to predict when ovulation will occur.

The mare can also be teased to show if she is in oestrus and willing to stand for the stallion. This is usually done with both the mare and stallion in hand but separated by a solid partition to protect the stallion from the mare, who has a tendency to become aggressive if she is not willing to stand. Some mares are particular about which stallions they will allow to cover them.

The mare ovulates about 48 hours before the end of oestrus, and if a mare is taken to a stallion it is usual for them to be mated on the second day of oestrus, and then every other day, until the mare will no longer stand. Ideally, the mare should be covered 12–24 hours before ovulation. This is because once the egg is shed it must be fertilized within about six hours, and sperm must be waiting for the egg before it is shed.

With artificial insemination it is often not possible to serve the mare frequently, because of the cost of sperm and the time for which it remains viable (sperm has only a limited 'life' once outside the stallion). Scanning is important to help achieve a successful mating.

The mare's oestrus cycle can also be manipulated hormonally to allow more accurate timing of ovulation and decrease the time of dioestrus and oestrus. The easiest way to bring a mare into oestrus quickly in the spring is to use artificial lighting in winter, to increase the hours of light to which she is exposed and so bring the seasonal cycling activity forward.

Pregnancy

The average pregnancy last between 330 and 345 days, but there is a wide variation, and many normal foals have been born at about 400 days!

Diagnosing pregnancy

Pregnancy should be confirmed as soon as possible, not only for interest but also to rule out the possibility of twins. The mare's placenta is not efficient enough to sustain twins to birth, and both twins are normally aborted at seven to eight months. If the twins survive until birth, they are normally weak and malformed and usually die soon after. There has been a very small number of normal live births of twins.

Suggested protocol for diagnosis

There are three principle stages at which the pregnancy is monitered:

First examination: At 14–15 days using ultrasound. This is the optimum time to confirm twins. If twins are found, it is possible to squeeze and remove one of the embryos.

Second examination: At 24–27 days using ultrasound to confirm twins. Twins can differ in age by to two or three days, so both are not always visible at 14–15 days. By day 26 it is possible to see a beating heart on the ultrasound scanner, and by day 28 it is possible for a vet to feel an embryo.

Third examination: At 33–35 days using manual palpation and ultrasound.

Blood tests can be used to confirm pregnancy in later stages because it is often difficult to manually palpate the foal, which may be deep in the abdomen.

Management of the pregnant mare

A number of elements contribute to the successful management of the pregnant mare:

- Adequate feeding.
- Proper parasite control; ivermectin at the normal dose rate to the mare in the last few days before foaling (or day of foaling) helps to prevent milk transfer of *Strongloides westeri* (threadworm).
- A clean, large stable, measuring at least 4 x 4m (13 x 13ft) for an average 500kg (1100lb) mare.

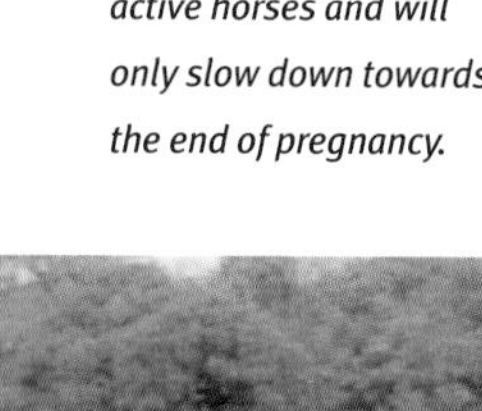

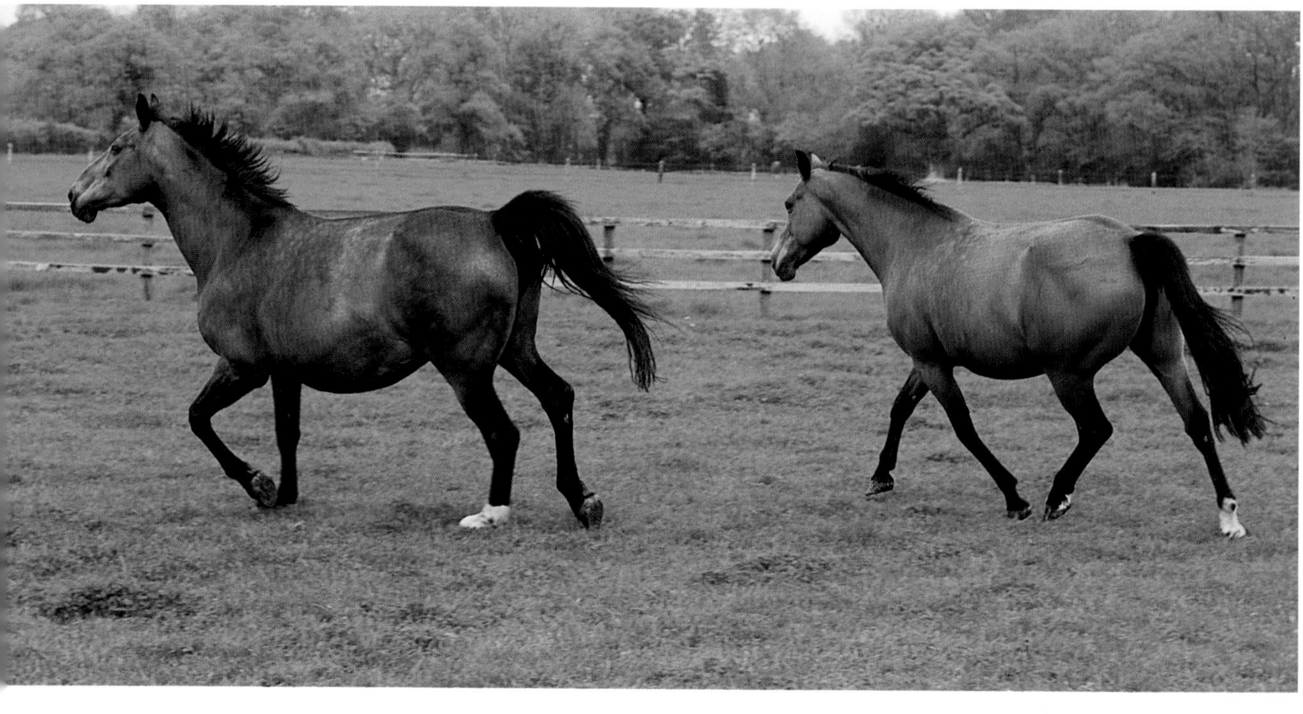

In-foal mares are still active horses and will only slow down towards the end of pregnancy.

Foaling

Foaling is a natural process and the vast majority of mares manage perfectly well unaided. However, if complications do arise it is vital that you are ready to contact the vet without delay.

A mare should be monitored closely in late pregnancy for the following physical changes, which are indicators for impending birth:

- Development of an udder
- Relaxation of the pelvic ligaments
- Lengthening of the vulva
- Swelling of the udder
- Waxing, a waxy excretion seen on the teat ends and leakage of colostrum; do not be tempted to keep pulling the teats to demonstrate that colostrum is present, as only a small amount is produced and the foal needs as much as possible

It is possible to measure the amount of calcium in the milk as a way of predicting foaling, but there is a significant risk to the foal in losing colostrum. There are also a number of foaling alarms available, which can be attached to the mare's vulva and are activated during straining or placed on her body and activated by sweating. Closed-circuit television can also be used.

Pre-foaling checks

Make sure that any caslick sutures have been removed and the vulva has been cut. Wash and dry the udder.

Stages of foaling

Mares do not like being watched or disturbed, and they will often put off labour until they are alone. The foaling process is commonly explained in three stages:

Stage 1: This begins with uterine contractions, which enable the foal to come into correct orientation in the pelvis. The clinical signs include restlessness, and the mare will often show colic-like signs (looking at the flank, tail twitching, constantly getting up and down), patchy sweating and yawning. At the end of first-stage labour, the sac surrounding the foal breaks (the waters break).

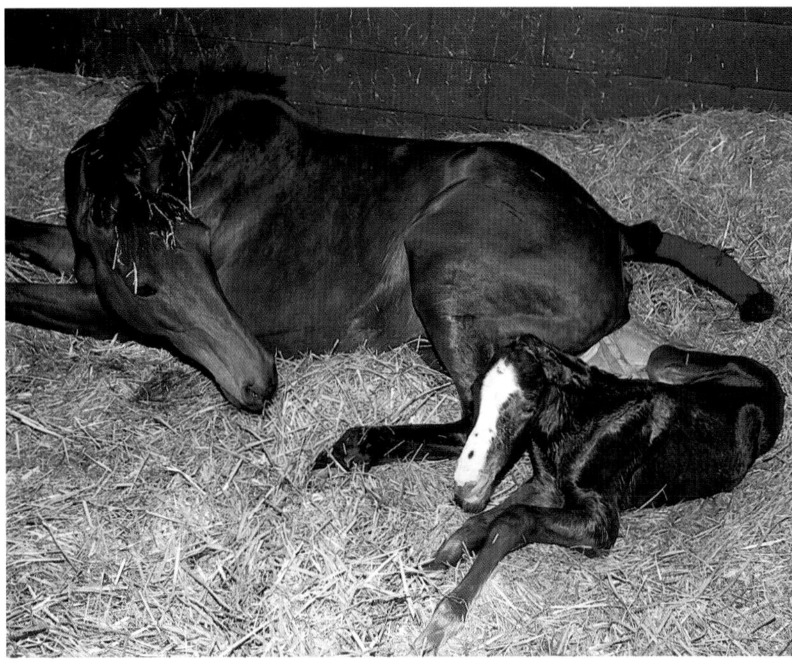

The hind feet of this newly born foal are still in the mare. However, within a couple of hours he will be standing on his own.

If possible, before the first stage of labour finishes a tail bandage should be applied and the vulva cleaned and dried. Have a bucket of warm water, some antiseptic and lubrication ready in case help is needed in the second stage.

Stage 2: This is indicated by the onset of abdominal straining and/or the appearance of a white, glistening sac (the amnion). The mare usually lies down and stays in lateral recumbency until the foal is born. Once the sac appears, a foot normally appears within five minutes, quickly followed by another foot, and then the nose. This stage of labour usually lasts about 15 minutes, and should not exceed one hour.

Once the foal has been born, do not cut the umbilicus. The foal is able to absorb up to 1.5 litres (2½ pints) of oxygenated blood from the mare after it has been born. The normal movements of the mare and foal will cause the umbilicus to break at a predisposed point about six to eight minutes after the actual

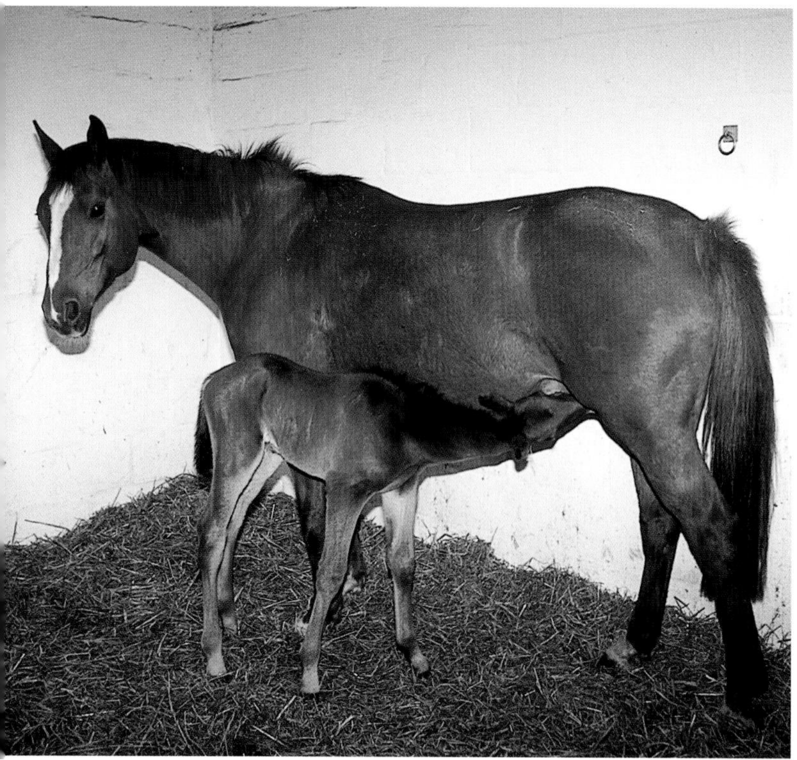

A newly born foal suckling from his mother.

birth. The umbilicus should then be disinfected or dipped in iodine. The foal can be pulled up to the head of the mare so that she doesn't stand on him, but try not to interfere.

Stage 3 This is the expulsion of the foetal membranes (afterbirth and placenta), which should take one to two hours. The membranes should be tied up to prevent the mare from standing on them. Veterinary advice should be sought if they have not been passed after two hours, because retained foetal membranes can make the mare very ill. In horses and ponies this tends to happen only after two or three days or more, but in large draught horses it can happen more quickly. If the membranes have not been passed, a vet will try a combination of manual removal and hormones (oxytocin) to try to get the mare to expel the membranes on her own. Antibiotics will also be given, both systemically (usually by an injection) and placed directly into the placenta.

Once the placenta has been passed, collect it so that it can be examined to make sure no bits have been left inside the mare.

Foaling problems

With any foaling problems, contact your vet as soon as possible – do not delay.

If nothing appears in the sac (the amnion) within five to ten minutes, veterinary advice should be sought immediately. This may mean that the foal is not presented correctly and will need to be manually re-oriented. Unlike cattle, there is only a very small amount of time available to correct these problems before the foal dies, so your vet may have to tell you what to do over the telephone.

If a red velvety sac appears at the vulva, contact the vet immediately. This usually means that the placenta is separating prematurely, effectively suffocating the foal as it will no longer be able to receive oxygenated blood from the umbilicus. Veterinary advice must be sought to confirm this, as it is possible to confuse it with prolapses (for example, rectal or bladder). If it is decided that the placenta has separated prematurely. then the sac must be broken and the foal delivered manually without delay.

Other problems where veterinary advice should be sought immediately are:

- Forced straining with nothing happening
- No straining for long periods once the sac has appeared
- Mare continually getting up and down
- The foal is stuck at the hips once the head, legs and chest are out
- Straining after the foetal membranes have been passed; this may indicate the presence of twins, a uterine or rectal tear.

Problems in the first 24 hours

A healthy foal is normally standing within one to three hours and should have sucked by two to four hours. Meconium, the black or brown material that has collected in the foal's intestine while in the womb, is usually passed without problems in the first 12–18 hours (24–36 hours maximum).

The umbilicus should be dipped or sprayed with disinfectant to help prevent infection. Ideally, the mare and foal should be checked by a vet in the first 24 hours to make sure the mare has no internal injuries or retained placenta, and to check the foal for congenital problems and give preventive tetanus antitoxin and sometimes antibiotics.

A newborn foal has a very poor immune system and relies on colostrum from the mare to provide him with antibodies to fight infection. It is, therefore, important that the foal receives adequate colostrum in the first 24 hours. Ideally, he should receive the colostrum within the first 12 hours, because his ability to absorb antibodies starts to decline after 24 hours. Between 3 and 4 litres (5–7 pints) are required in the first 24 hours.

Symptoms Not standing, difficulty breathing, bent legs, colic, milk pouring from nose when suckling.

Causes

- **Not standing:** This may be because the foal is too weak, indicating a difficult birth, or due to brain damage caused by lack of oxygen. It may also be neonatal maladjustment syndrome (also known as barkers, wanderers or dummies). He could be a premature foal, have fractures in the pelvis or limbs caused by a difficult birth, or flexed or contracted limbs.
- **Difficulty breathing:** This can be common in premature foals, which do not have enough of a specialized liquid, surfactant, in their lungs to enable them to fill with air. It may be associated with breathing in meconium while still inside the mare.
- **Bent legs:** This may be caused by excessive contraction of the flexor tendons or deformities in the limbs.
- **Colic:** This may be caused by retained meconium, an abnormally developed gastro-intestinal tract or a ruptured bladder, which can occur during foaling.
- **Milk pouring from nose:** This is commonly associated with a cleft palate. Foals are also susceptible to aspiration pneumonia, which must be checked for quickly.

DIAGNOSIS

A full clinical examination will be necessary, together any history of foaling problems, recent illness or problems with the mare before foaling.

Owner action Keep notes related to the foaling. Did the foal ever stand? When did the colic start? Was the foal premature?

Treatment Treatment depends on the cause. Ill foals require urgent and intensive treatment. Foals with flexed legs may be given intravenous treatment with oxytetracycline. Many problems will improve within 48 hours, but after that further treatment for foal orthopaedic problems (see page 109) may be needed.

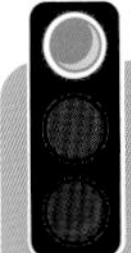

URGENCY INDICATOR

Very urgent.

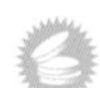

COST

Intensive nursing of the foal, even before any treatment, is very expensive.

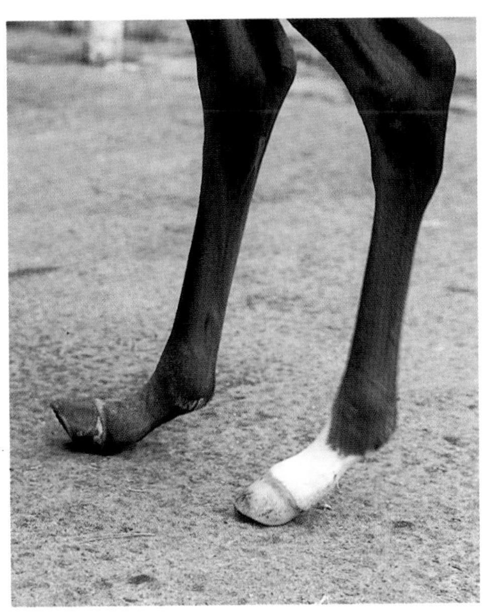

This foal is suffering from bent legs caused by flexor tendon laxity.

Problems after 24 hours

Although the first 24 hours are the most critical, unfortunately there is still a high risk of potential problems in the following weeks.

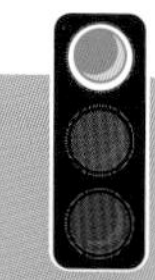

URGENCY INDICATOR

Very urgent.

COST

Intensive nursing is very expensive.

Symptoms Bent legs (see page 107) or extended legs (see page 109), progressive lethargy, fitting, anaemia, temperature, diarrhoea, nasal discharge, cough.

Causes Failure to get enough colostrum in first 24 hours predisposes the foal to infection; infection from the umbilicus; neonatal isoethryrolysis syndrome, a condition in which the antibodies absorbed by the foal through colostrum actually destroy the foal's red blood cells; bacterial or viral infections, which may be caused by inadequate colostrum intake in the first 24 hours; foal heat (diarrhoea).

Owner action Know the mare's history. Has she been vaccinated? Know the mare's previous foaling history and monitor the foal closely. How much colostrum did the foal have? Did the mare leak colostrum before foaling?

DIAGNOSIS

Full clinical examination and blood and antibody tests will be carried out. X-rays may be used if there are respiratory problems.

Treatment Treatment will depend on the condition. In cases of neonatal isoethryrolysis syndrome, the foal will need to be separated from the mare until she has stopped producing colostrum and will require blood transfusions and intensive nursing. Foals with no immunity will require hyper-immune serum transfusions, antibiotics and supportive nursing.

Diarrhoea between one and two weeks is often called 'foal heat' diarrhoea. It is caused by the foal being naturally coprophagic (eating his own faeces) and establishing the normal bacteria in the gastro-intestinal tract. If the foal is well and does not have a temperature, treatment is often not needed. Alternatively, a binding agent, such as kaolin, can be used. The diarrhoea is not caused by the mare being in season, as is often thought. If the foal is ill or has a temperature, antibiotics and possibly supportive nursing are required. Respiratory infections will require antibiotics.

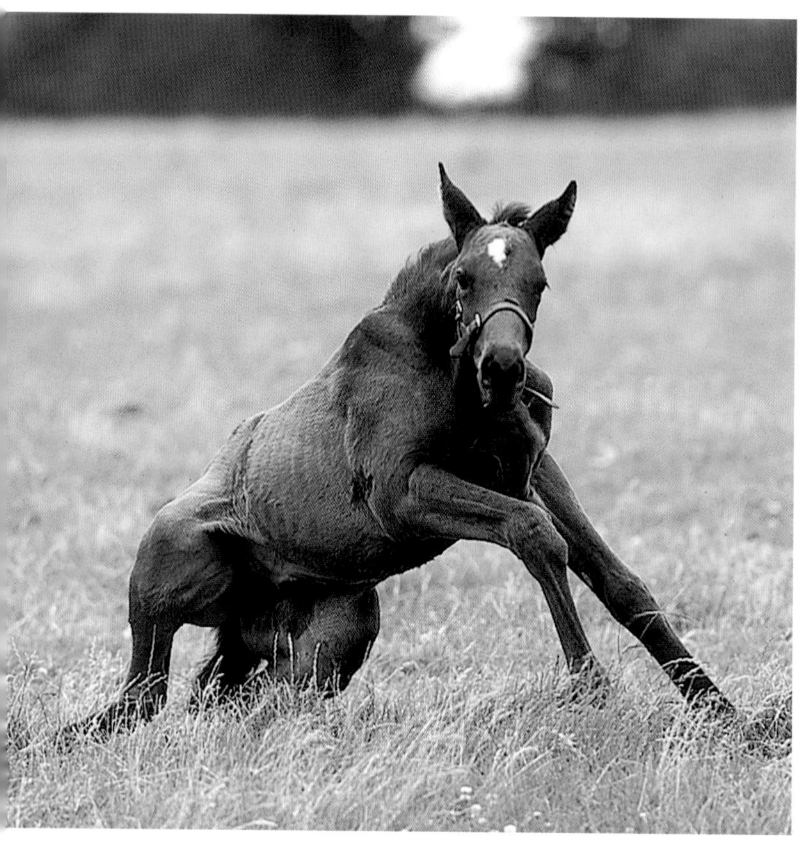

The proportionally long legs that give foals their appealing appearance can cause them problems in standing and moving if they have birth deformities.

Care of the older foal

Foals should be handled as much as possible. Get them used to being touched so that, for example, they are happy to pick their feet up when asked. This makes examining older foals easier and safer if they have any problems.

Feet

The foal's feet should be checked from two months onwards by a farrier.

Worming

Foals should be wormed from six to eight weeks of age, then at eight-week intervals with ivermectin until they are six months old, then every eight to ten weeks. Benzimadazoles can be used from about six weeks, although they can also be used therapeutically against threadworm at three weeks of age. Pyrantel can be used in foals over four weeks of age.

Foal worms

Threadworms (*Strongyloides westeri*), can be transmitted from mare to foal in the milk. Prevention involves giving ivermectin at the normal rate to the mare in the last few days before foaling or even on the day of foaling. Infection can cause diarrhoea and unthriftiness in the foal.

Roundworms (*Parascaris equorum*), are transmitted from foal to foal in successive years on the pasture. Treatment every six weeks in the foal's first grazing season helps to prevent infection.

Ideally, foals with mares should be grazed on pasture that was not grazed by foals in the previous year. Once weaned, foals and yearlings should be kept away from adult stock. They should never graze on pasture after adults have grazed it in the pasture rotation.

Vaccination

This should be done from about six months.

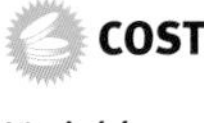

COST

Variable.

Orthopaedic problems

Due to the fact that foals have proportionally long legs, problems with their tendons and joints are very common.

Symptoms Difficulty standing, over-flexed or over-extended legs (flexural limb deformities), bent legs (angular limb deformities), lameness and swelling over joints (joint ill, osteochondrosis, physitis).

Causes Most limb deformities, except for those obviously caused by either trauma or infection, are developmental problems, which can have many different causes and often more than one. Common factors include genetics, rapid growth, hormonal disturbances, trauma and nutrition.

Owner action Many developmental problems may be associated with feeding too much to the foal or mare. Ask your vet about changing the feeding regime.

DIAGNOSIS

This will involve taking a thorough history and determining if the foal was born like this, and/or when it started to occur. If relevant, X-rays will be taken to assess the development of the bones. Sometimes arthroscopy will be necessary.

Treatment This will depend on the cause. Flexural and angular limb deformities may be treated with a combination of splints or plastic glue-on shoes with extensions. As a last resort, it may be necessary to correct some of the deformities surgically, either by tendon surgery or bone pinning, to allow even growth. Nutritional supplements, such as chondroitin, glucosamine and MSM, may be used to improve the joints.

URGENCY INDICATOR

Urgent.

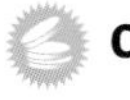

COST

Variable.

The competition horse

The competition horse suffers from the same types of problem as other riding horses, but there are the added factors of the stress of the particular competition field in which he is expected to perform. The higher the level at which the horse performs, the more intense are the stresses of that particular sport. For example, the complex movements performed by the dressage horse place considerable stress on the joints and tendons of the lower limbs. The hock joint, for instance, will be put under intense stress by piaffe, which involves a certain amount of abnormal loading. In the jumping horse the hock joint is put under stress, which increases with the level at which the horse performs. In addition, the forelimbs of jumping horses suffer extra stress on landing, and the tendons, check ligaments and suspensory ligaments come under particular pressure. In the racehorse the flexor tendons are especially prone to damage. This sports horse is performing at maximum pressure during each race, and if muscular tiring occurs extra stress and pressure are placed on the tendons.

These are just a few of the ways in which particular types of competition place stress on individual horses. There are obviously ways to avoid the common problems that arise from competition, and these are discussed in this section. They do not necessarily apply with equal importance to each sporting discipline, but it is always vital to prepare and protect your horse before any performance in any type of competitive activity.

Before, during and after competition

Having spent a great deal of time and expense getting your competition horse fit, it is only sensible to limit potential problems by careful pre-planning and preparation.

Vaccinations

Vaccines provide important protection against diseases such as flu and herpes, which are common risks at competition venues. Never forget the importance of tetanus vaccination, because small, penetrative wounds can cause this fatal disease. Remember to consider rabies vaccination if you are competing in a country where this disease is endemic. Check that your horse's documentation is correct and that all vaccinations required for competition are entered into it.

Fitness

The importance of fitness before and during competition cannot be over-emphasized and must be monitored during competition. Monitoring your horse's respiration, pulse and temperature at the same time of day and at the same stage of your exercise programme each time is very important.

Remember to examine your horse before and after competition, paying particular attention to the lower limbs. Carry out a visual inspection followed by a manual palpation of the lower limb. Do not forget to remove all bandages for an hour before monitoring limbs.

Blood sampling for health checks on a regular basis before and after competition can be useful, but remember that you need a base line for your particular horse, and a single sample is not always of great significance.

Nutrition

Monitoring fluid intake before, during and after competition is essential. This is easily done by using graduated water buckets or a measuring stick, which can be put into the bucket before it is refilled. Never restrict your horse's access to water and make sure that the water is palatable, by using water filters if necessary. The idea that water should be restricted before a competition is a fallacy, and there is no harm in letting your horse drink a small

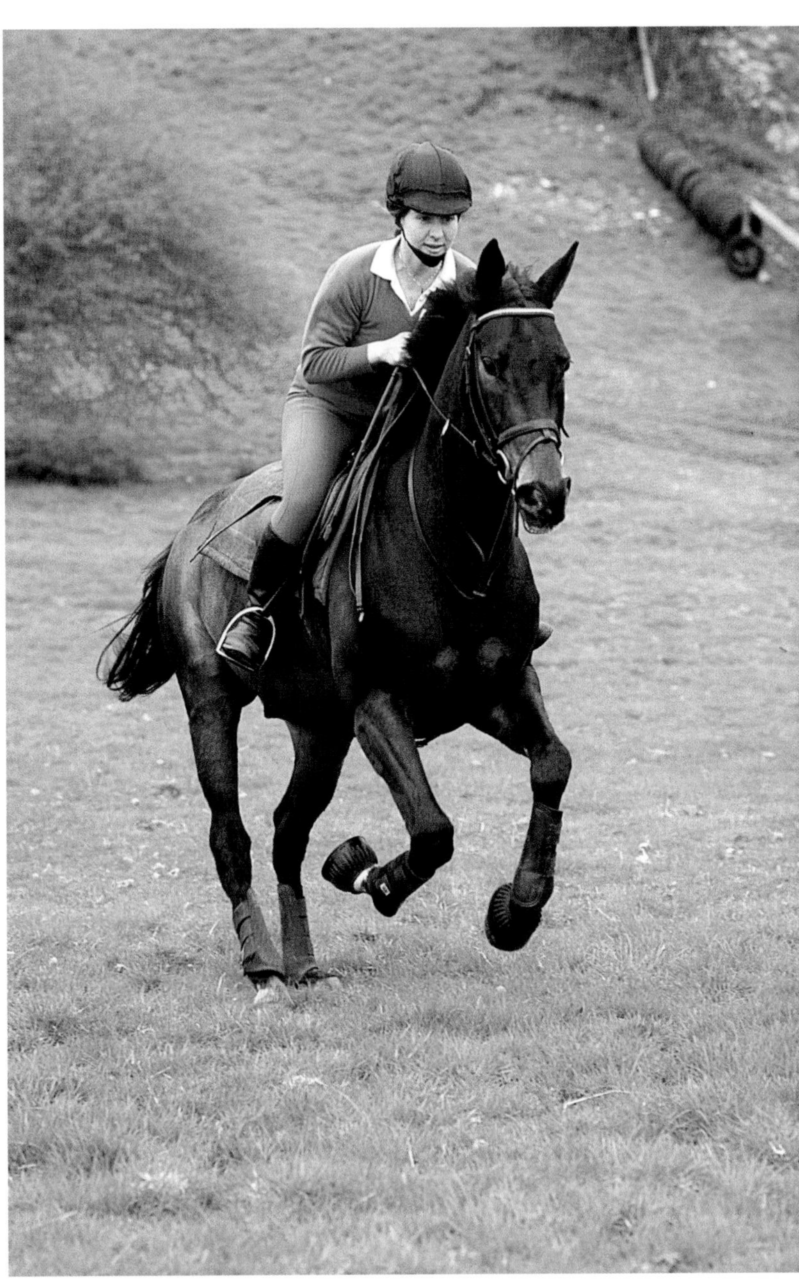

Regular exercise to ensure that the horse is fit is the most important part of the preparation for any competition.

amount of water during competition, for example in the ten-minute box in the three-day-event, between rounds in show jumping or during long warm-up periods in dressage. Drinking helps to cool the horse down and prevents dehydration.

Food intake must be carefully monitored. It is important not to change feeds during competition, and it is useful to take your own feed with you. The type of feeds required will depend on the demands made by the particular type of competition.

When bandaging the horse's legs it is important to make sure that the bandage is neither too tight nor too loose.

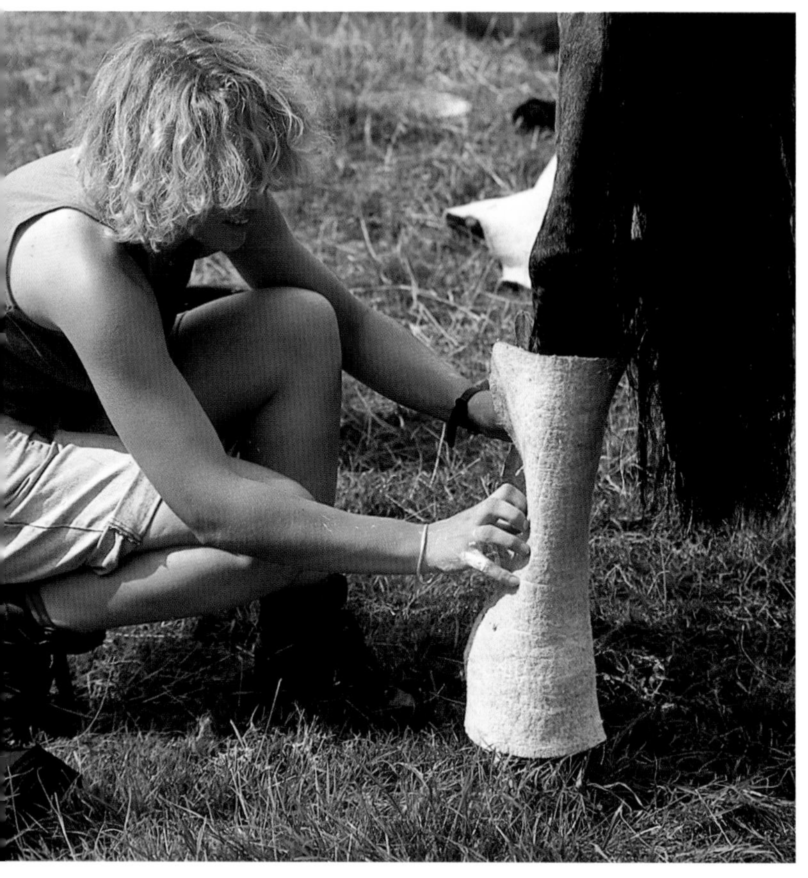

Shoeing

Well-balanced, well-shod horses perform better and sustain fewer injuries. They also have a longer working life. Shoe at least seven to ten days before the competition to avoid nail bind, pricks or soreness from feet being cut back. Never compete if the shoes need replacing or the feet need trimming. Check feet and shoes regularly both before and after competition.

Carry spare sets of shoes, studs and nails of the correct size if you are travelling away from home. If studs are used, they should be bilateral (in both heels) to prevent any twisting that using a single stud may create. Carry equipment for emergency shoe removal and make sure you know how to use it. Boots to protect the foot on a temporary basis are available and are also useful as an emergency poultice boot.

Bandaging

There is much debate about the use and value of bandaging, but when used both bandages and boots must be carefully adjusted and checked regularly during exercise to prevent slippage and constriction of the blood supply to the limbs.

Protecting the horse in competitions

Making sure your horse is correctly kitted out is essential in any competition:

Saddlery: A well-fitted saddle and bridle are extremely important, both for the physical well-being of the horse and for the safety of the rider. Always carry spares and always check them before and after competition. Make sure the contact areas are kept extremely clean. Many modern materials, such as gel pads and new materials for saddlecloths and numnahs, help to protect your horse.

Leg protection: Bandages and boots have little part to play in reducing strain but can be useful in protecting lower limbs and joints from impact. The correct fitting of boots and bandages is critical. There must be no mud and sand between the boot and the skin. Over-loose or over-tight boots and bandages can slip or constrict and cause long-term damage to the horse's legs.

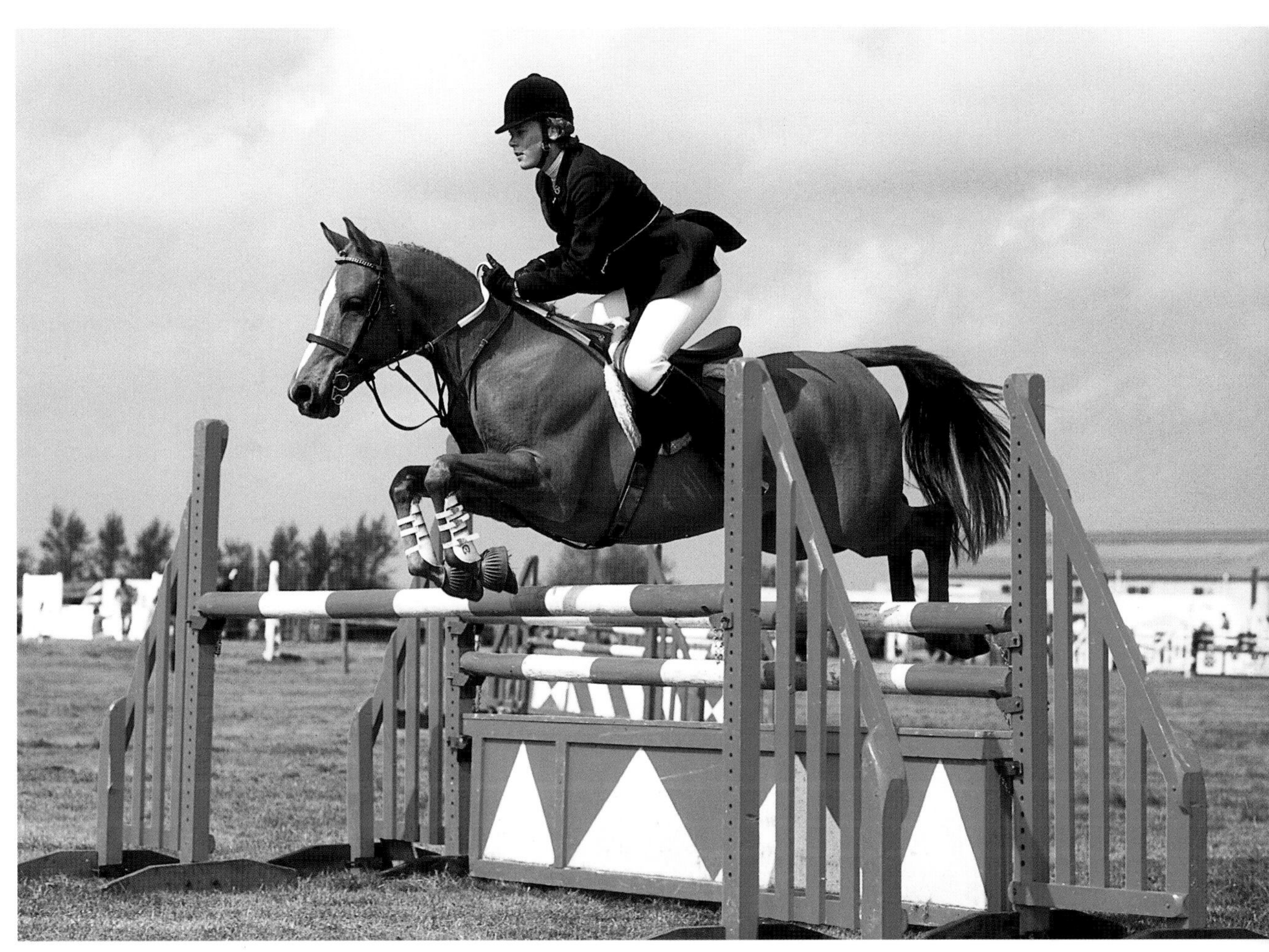

Environment

During travel and when your horse is in unfamiliar stables and show grounds, he may be exposed to unsatisfactory and dusty environments. Try to protect your horse as much as you can because respiratory conditions are very common, and it would be a disaster to have prepared a horse that cannot perform because of a last-minute response to dust. Take dust-free hay or haylage and dampen all your feeds. Making sure the bedding is dust-free helps to produce a good atmosphere. Adequate ventilation both during transport and in the stable is extremely important. Finally, remember that although the stable your horse is in may be dust-free, the boxes around you may not be, so try to protect your horse from this as much as possible.

After the competition has finished, it is important to check your horse for any minor injuries while you are washing him down. Make sure he cools down slowly, and also ensure that there is plenty of water available so that rehydration can take place.

Jumping puts considerable stress on the horse's legs so good protection is vital.

+ First aid

The most important aspect of first aid is **safety**. You must not put yourself or any other person into a situation where you or they may be hurt. Even the most placid horse may behave unpredictably when in pain, because he will be confused and frightened. Before you examine your horse, make sure that he is securely restrained by someone competent. Try to keep the horse calm and do not leave him alone, unless there is no alternative.

First aid is just that – the immediate help that you give your horse before the vet gets there. You should avoid doing anything that will prevent your vet doing what he needs to – for example, don't put antiseptic cream or antibacterial sprays on wounds that may need stitching.

It is always best to apply clean, preferably sterile, dressings to wounds, but if you don't have any to hand use the cleanest suitable alternative, such as a clean disposable nappy. Slowing down the bleeding is important at this point; the wound can always be sterilized again. Do not use anything fluffy that might shed bits into the wound or anything that might adhere.

FIRST AID KIT

A basic first aid kit should contain the items listed below. Keep it close at hand at all times and take it with you whenever you transport your horse anywhere. Always replace any item you use straight away, before it is needed again.

- blunt-ended curved scissors
- sterile non-stick dressings
- stretchy, adhesive and soft bandages
- gauze-covered cotton wool, such as veterinary gamgee
- waterproof bandage tape
- salt to add to water for washing wounds
- chlorhexidine or iodine
- clear wound-packing gel, such as aloe vera gel
- wound cream
- wound spray
- equine thermometer
- poultice

Wounds

Call the vet as soon as possible for any wound that will need stitching. The sooner it is stitched, the better. Cells at the edge of wounds start to die almost immediately, and after just six or seven hours your vet will have to trim back skin and muscle in order to be able to set stitches and stretch the muscle and skin.

If there is excessive bleeding, apply pressure to the wound using a sterile dressing. If an artery in a limb is injured, apply a tourniquet above the wound, but slacken off the pressure briefly every ten minutes so that the blood supply to the rest of the limb is not cut off completely.

Then clean the wound, gently. Do not try to pick out foreign bodies as you may break them, leaving shorter pieces that will be difficult to remove. Gently wash warm salty water over small wounds to clean and disinfect them. Use one teaspoon of salt to 600ml (20fl oz/1 pint) of water. Using too strong a disinfectant solution may actually kill off skin cells, so avoid this.

If the wound is very large, clean it with water from a hose (see opposite) and disinfect it with salty water. Cooling down the area of the wound with water also helps to minimize any swelling.

If the wound is deep, pack it with clear, wound-packing gel according to the instructions on the packet, then cover it with a sterile dressing until veterinary assistance arrives. Do not apply wound cream or spray to the area until a vet has examined the wound, as this may prevent the wound from being stitched if required.

Pad the area of the wound with gauze cotton wool or gamgee, and then wrap it with a support bandage to minimize further swelling.

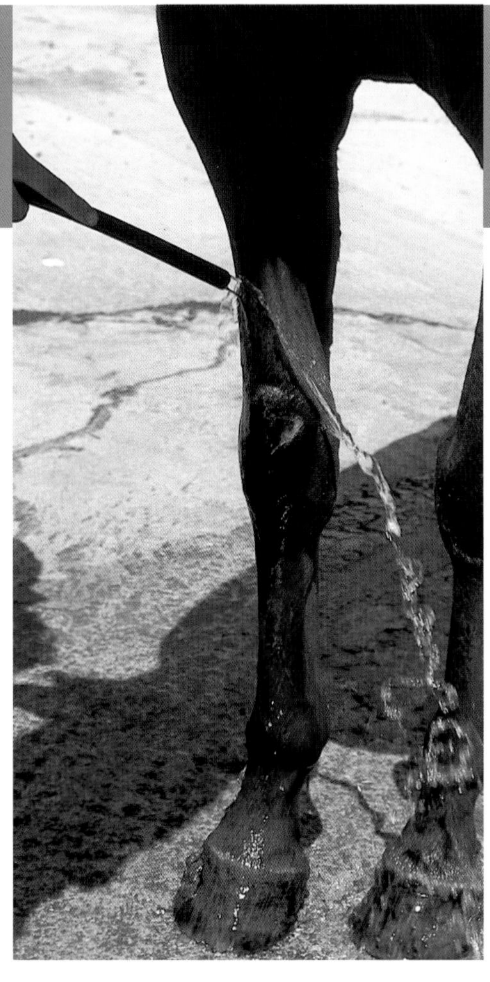

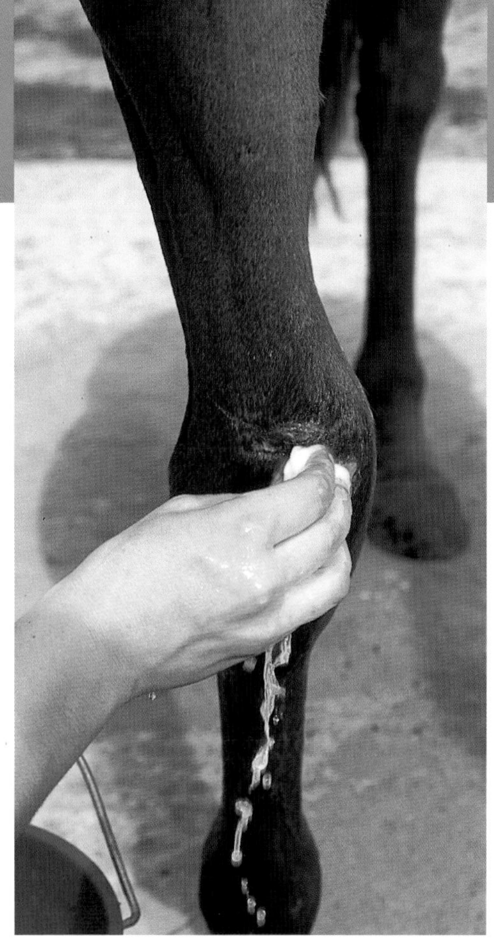

far left: To clean a large wound, slowly run water from a hose over it.

left: Clean the wound with salty water, then gently dry it with a sterile pad.

Fractures

If you suspect that your horse has fractured a leg, splint it and keep the horse as still as possible until the vet arrives.

Burns

Wash the wound with cold water for at least ten minutes – using a hose is the easiest method. Do not put anything on the burn until it has been seen by the vet.

Chemical burns

Seek veterinary advice immediately. If the chemical is dry, brush it off with a soft brush; otherwise, wash all contaminated areas with as much water as possible. Be careful not to contaminate yourself.

Sunburn

Bare patches of pink skin, for example the nose, can get sunburned. Cool the area with cold water, then apply a soothing, non-oily cream.

Bites and stings

Apply a cold compress to the sting to help reduce any inflammation. If the sting is very painful, call your vet, who will be able to prescribe anti-inflammatories.

Foreign objects penetrating the foot

Leave any object penetrating the foot in place, so that the vet can assess the angle and depth of the wound. If left untreated, damage to any of the many underlying tissues in the hoof could result in permanent lameness.

Tendon swellings

Any swellings in areas with tendons (see page 76) or accompanied by lameness should be examined by a vet. Hose down the affected limb with cold water for at least ten minutes, dry off and apply a stable bandage (see page 116) to prevent further swelling. To provide further support for the injured leg, apply stable bandages to the other legs as well.

WARNING

Your vet should examine any wound overlying a joint or tendon to make sure that none of the tissues under the skin have been damaged.

Dehydration

In hot weather or while working, horses lose large amounts of fluid from their breathing surfaces, and if this is not replenished they will become dehydrated. They can also become dehydrated as a result of diarrhoea or some forms of poisoning. If you notice that your horse has dull, sunken eyes, is breathing rapidly or shallowly, or even panting, he is not sweating or urinating, or has dark urine and his faeces are dry (except in the case of diarrhoea), he is not getting enough fluids. An easy way to tell if a horse is dehydrated is to pinch a small fold of skin. If it stays up rather than springing back flat as soon as you release it, your horse is dehydrated.

It is imperative to get fluid into your horse as quickly as possible by giving him as much water to drink as he wants. To replace any salts that may have been lost, add an electrolyte mixture to the water. In an emergency, where you do not have any electrolytes, add salt to the water: 30g to every 5 litres (1oz to 9 pints) is sufficient. Any treatment must be continued until the horse is no longer dehydrated: in the case of diarrhoea, this may be some days.

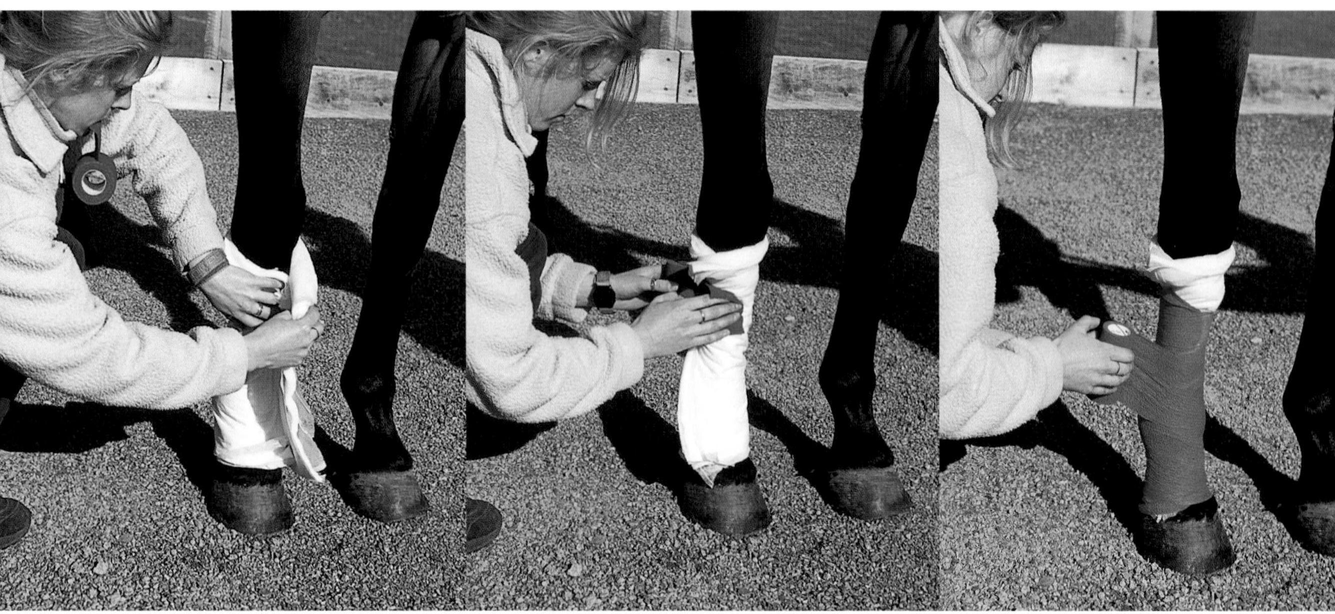

1 *The most important thing to remember in bandaging is padding. If in doubt, add more. If a dressing is required, hold this is place with a soft co-forming bandage, rather than an elasticated bandage which is not designed to go directly on the skin and can cause bandage sores.*

2 *Apply a covering of cotton wool, gamgee or synthetic bandage padding. This can be held in place with an elasticated bandage or fastened at the top and bottom with elastoplast to prevent slipping. This will also help to prevent debris, such as shavings, getting into the bandage.*

3 *When applying the bandage, unroll it a little first so that it is not applied under too much tension. Always bandage away from you, starting at the back of the leg and coming inside the leg to the front. Apply the bandage evenly, with approximately one third overlap on each layer.*

Acute emergencies

Collapse

Horses collapse for a variety of reasons. Among the most common are colic (see pages 44–45), EHV1 infection (see page 90), poisoning, spinal cord trauma, exhaustion, fractured pelvis or femur, and nettle stings.

The first thing to do is to make sure that your horse's airway is clear, by straightening his head and neck carefully and removing any obvious obstructions. Check whether the horse is breathing and has a pulse, then telephone the vet immediately.

Keep your horse warm until veterinary attention arrives. Be very careful near his legs as horses can be very unpredictable, and obey all the usual rules about not spooking him. Try to ascertain how long your horse has been down and what he was doing before he collapsed. Check to see whether there are any obvious wounds, bites, stings or fractures, and check his mouth to see whether he might have eaten something poisonous (see page 122). Details like this will help the vet to make an accurate diagnosis and start appropriate treatment as quickly as possible.

Severe distress

An extremely agitated horse, often with saliva pouring from his nose, or showing signs of colic, is severely distressed.

The underlying causes of severe distress include the following:

- **Choke** If you suspect that your horse is suffering from choke (see page 43), you should remove all food immediately. If your horse has been feeding recently, choke is very likely, and if you suspect that is the case massage the left side of his neck, from the top to the base in long, sweeping movements. Choke will often clear on its own in 15–20 minutes. Longer periods of choke always require veterinary assistance to remove the obstruction. It is often advisable to get the horse endoscoped to check for damage to the oesophagus following choke.
- **Colic** Remove all food from the horse's reach. If he is stabled, remove any edible bedding and replace it with a non-edible variety. Bank this up the edges of the stable, so that if your horse lies down or falls he will be able to get a grip in the bedding and

TAKING A HORSE'S TEMPERATURE

The 'normal' temperature for a horse is 37.7–38.5°C (99.5–101.5°F). If your horse's temperature is above this range, call the vet immediately.

1 Digital thermometers are best for this. If possible, tie a piece of string to the back end of the thermometer so that you can retrieve it more easily if it disappears.

2 Make sure that the horse is restrained, especially if he is not used to having his temperature taken.

3 If you are using a mercury thermometer, shake the mercury down to below 37.7°C (99.5°F), or lower if you know your horse usually has a lower-than-average temperature.

4 Put on a pair of surgical gloves, lubricate the business end of the thermometer, run your hand over the horse's quarters so that you don't surprise him and lift his tail. Make sure you are standing to one side and not within reach of his hoof.

5 Gently push the thermometer into the horse's rectum (just over halfway for mercury thermometers and according to the instructions for digital thermometers).

6 Leave the thermometer in place for two minutes, withdraw it gently, wipe it off and then check the reading.

7 Remember to disinfect the thermometer (use cold water, not hot) after you have finished.

get back up. Contact the vet without delay, even if the symptoms (see pages 44–45) are not severe.

- **Strangles** If you suspect that your horse has strangles (see page 55) because he is making strangled breathing noises, call the vet immediately – the sooner the horse is started on a course of antibiotics, the more likely he is to recover.
- **Upper respiratory tract obstruction** An obstruction can be caused by an abscess or foreign bodies in the pharynx, a swelling associated with a reaction to a bite or sting or a reaction to a drug. Keep the horse's neck extended and seek veterinary attention immediately. In extreme cases, an emergency tracheotomy may need to be performed to remove the obstruction.

KNOW YOUR HORSE'S BASELINE SIGNS

If you know your horse's normal baseline signs for resting pulse rate, temperature and breathing rate, you can spot more easily if there is something wrong. For example, 35 heartbeats a minute is well within normal limits for horses, but if you know your horse's normal resting pulse rate is 28, it may be an indication that there is a problem.

CHECKING YOUR HORSE'S PULSE AND BREATHING RATES

Most horses have a resting pulse rate of 30–40 beats per minute, although this varies between individuals and increases with exercise. Check your horse's pulse rate by holding one finger (not thumb) flat against the artery that runs under the jaw. If you know your horse's normal pulse rate, you can spot whether there may be something wrong more easily. A normal resting breathing rate for a horse is roughly 12–20 breaths per minute. Shallow, rapid breaths may indicate shock, and ragged breathing is usually an indication of pain.

Trailer or lorry accidents

If you are involved in an accident with a trailer or a lorry the first and most important thing is to check for human casualties, make sure no-one else gets hurt and call the emergency services if necessary (if anyone is injured or the vehicle is causing an obstruction). If possible, try to calm the horse by talking to him and reassuring him, but do not get into the lorry or trailer – you may spook him further and a frightened horse may cause damage to you as well as it himself. If possible, remove any objects on which he may further hurt himself, but not if doing so would frighten the animal.

When the vet arrives, he will be able to assess any injuries to the horse and the best course of action. Normally horses need to be sedated before they can be moved, to prevent further injury not only to themselves but also to any people. This also applies if a horse has gone through the floor of a trailer. If the horse is not hurt or too stressed it may be possible for him to climb out of the floor, but if you are in any doubt, keep him calm and wait for veterinary assistance.

Treating stiffness and strains

Physiotherapy, myotherapy (muscle therapy), sports massage and physical therapy can all be used to treat problems in the muscles, joints, tendons, ligaments and other support structures of the horse.

There are a number of stages in the diagnosis and treatment:

- diagnose the problem and its cause
- remove the cause of the problem, if possible
- treat both the specific problem and the whole horse
- follow-up therapy

It is important to remember that a horse functions as a unit: the health and efficiency of one part of his body directly affects those of its neighbouring parts. When one part is in pain or not working properly, it causes extra stress on other parts of the body, which then develop pain and stop working efficiently in turn. Any condition that causes a change, however slight, in a horse's motion will lead to compensation and, as a result, pain throughout different parts of the body. If, for example, the horse has pain in one leg, he will change his movement to favour that leg. He may then develop muscle soreness and pain in the opposing limb, and particularly in the back and neck through extra stress being placed on them. To cure the horse, or at least alleviate the problem as much as possible, his whole body must be treated, not just what appears to be the most obvious or immediate complaint at the time. This is often called holistic (whole-body) medicine.

Symptoms of pain in horses

There are a variety of symptoms, some of which are physical and some behavioural. You may notice them when riding, working, grooming or tacking up.

Physical symptoms:

- lameness, dragging feet or stumbling
- stiffness when working on one rein

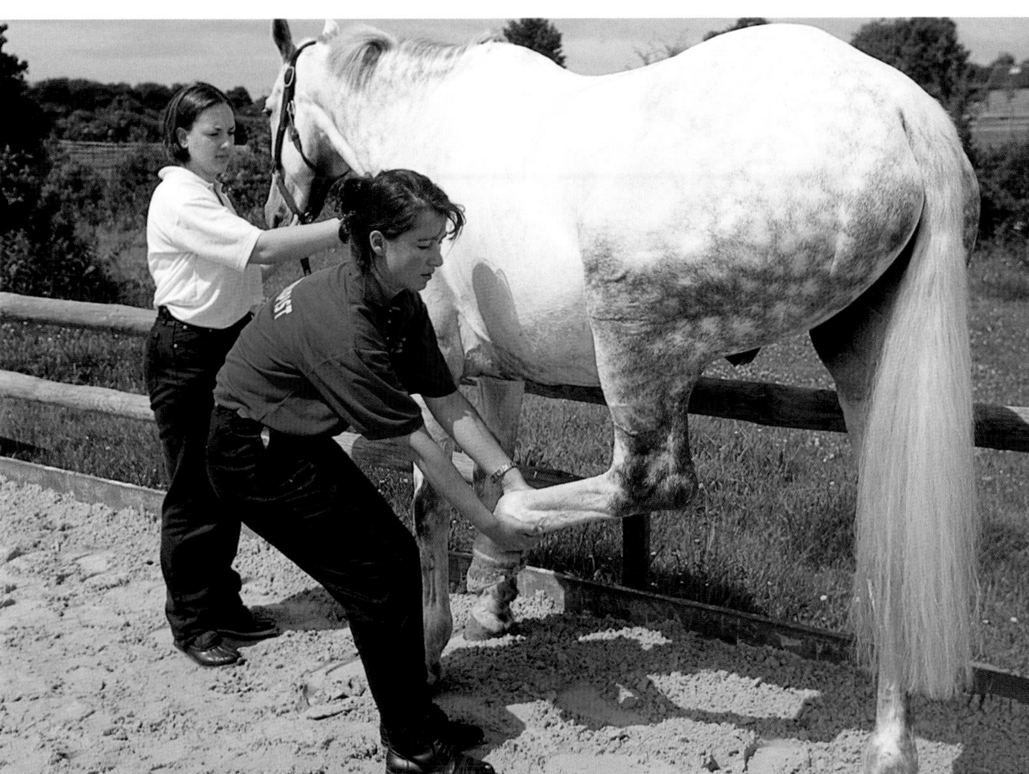

Physiotherapy can be used to treat a wide range of problems.

- hitting jumps with front or rear feet or legs
- not feeling normal when ridden, uncomfortable when changing paces
- noticeable difference in feel when changing diagonals at trot
- tight, hard muscle when touched
- heat or pain when muscles touched
- abnormal swelling or hard lumps of tissue within muscles
- uneven muscle development on one side compared to the other
- muscles that have not built up with work or lack tone
- sore (cold) back

Behavioural symptoms:

- napping when working, or when you are doing up his girth or putting on his saddle
- bucking or rearing
- resistance when asked to do particular forms of work or movements – for example, putting his ears back, kicking out or generally being unhappy
- depression, aggression or unhappiness
- laziness when hacking, or at the start of a ride, then warming up after 10–15 minutes
- lack of appetite

Common causes of muscle soreness

- **Ill-fitting tack** Saddles, especially, can cause severe muscle soreness and the behavioural symptoms described above if they are not properly fitted. There are qualified saddle fitters in most areas – ask your vet for advice. All saddles should be checked regularly to make sure they fit correctly, because if your horse has gained weight or built up more muscle the saddle will be tight or ill-fitting, and over time this can cause a lot of damage and pain.
- **Injuries** Falling over, slipping, getting cast in the stable, scrambling and falling over in the lorry/trailer or direct trauma. Any incident in which the horse has suffered damage to the muscles can cause bleeding within them and straining of the muscle fibres. This will cause heat and pain, and needs to be treated to avoid scar tissue and resulting problems. Often the horse is sore or lame and you can feel swellings or heat in the area, or your horse will be reluctant to let you touch it.
- **Incorrect shoeing** If the horse has foot pain as a result of underlying problems or incorrect farriery, then this can cause soreness of the muscles of the shoulder, withers or neck area (in the case of the front feet) or the lower back and rump area (if his back feet are affected).
- **Abrupt change in workload or type of work** Any change in workload or type of work should be gradual to build up the appropriate muscles. If the transition is too fast, it will result in tight, sore muscles. Over time, the cumulative effects of this will cause loss of ease of motion and a range of behavioural symptoms. Racehorses or horses with a heavy competition schedule can develop stiff, tight muscles because of stresses placed on them on a regular basis. Ongoing treatment can help to decrease the recovery time needed after events and help the horse to attain optimum performance levels.
- **Rider imbalance** If the rider is unbalanced or perhaps has had an injury, this can place uneven weight on the horse, which will cause uneven muscle build-up and imbalance within the horse's action. If you do not ensure that you are riding correctly, this can cause soreness and a change in overall motion of the horse.

If you suspect your horse is muscle sore or stiff and think he may benefit from treatment, the first thing to do is to ring your vet. There is nothing to gain by not treating the underlying causes; if just the muscle soreness is treated, it

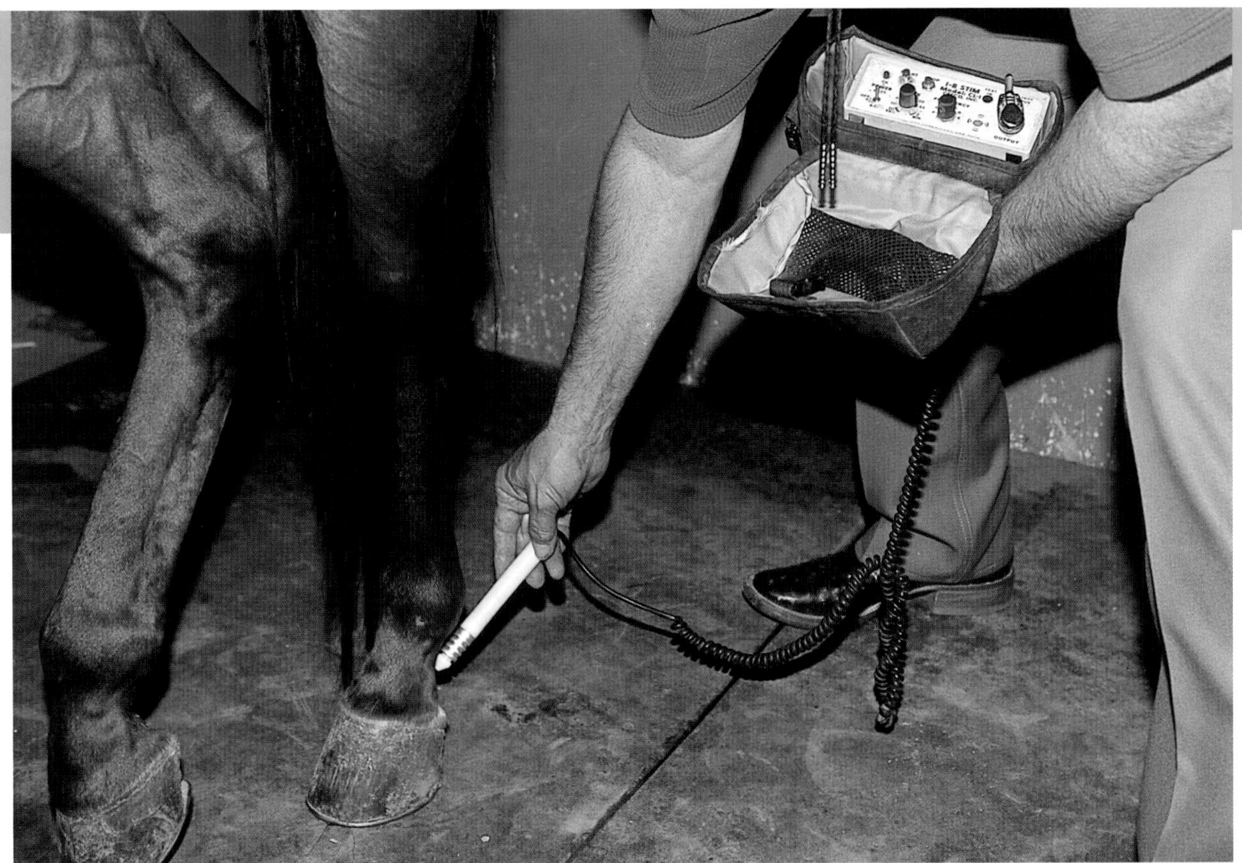

will simply recur. If there are no underlying causes, the vet will work with your therapist to decide on the appropriate treatment. Then a protocol is worked out – usually involving a slight adjustment to work, some different exercises and some stretching, all of which will involve some time and dedication by you to get your horse back on track. Often the co-operation of the saddle fitter, farrier and trainer are also required to ensure there is a holistic assessment and approach. If symptoms are ignored, then you can actually cause a lot of damage with continued work.

Treatment

Various forms of physiotherapy, including ultrasound, laser treatment and heat therapy, can be used on the main sites of pain, as well as alternative therapies, such as acupressure, acupuncture and magnetic therapy. In the early stages after an injury, physiotherapy is used to improve localized blood flow, which helps to remove heat, pain and bruising from the area, encourage tissue repair and minimize scarring. It also helps to reduce scar tissue in older injuries.

Treating muscle soreness

If your horse has had a recent injury, is uncomfortable, has any abnormal swellings and is not eating or is depressed, call the vet immediately. Recent muscle injuries may need treatment for anything up to 10–14 days after the initial healing process begins.

The usual approach to muscle soreness is hands-on treatment directly on the muscles with massage and deep tissue therapy, accompanied by a wide range of stretching and exercises to help build up the muscles again. Often in long-standing cases the original cause of the compensation may have gone, but the restriction of movement acquired when the horse was compensating remains and this must be treated. Massage and exercise can help rebalance the whole horse by releasing tight muscles, restoring flexibility and stopping this 'protective splinting syndrome'. Massage and exercise also generally increase the fitness and vitality of your horse.

Laser treatment is used to improve blood flow in the area of a wound and thus reduce inflammation, heat and pain, and to promote tissue growth.

Poisoning

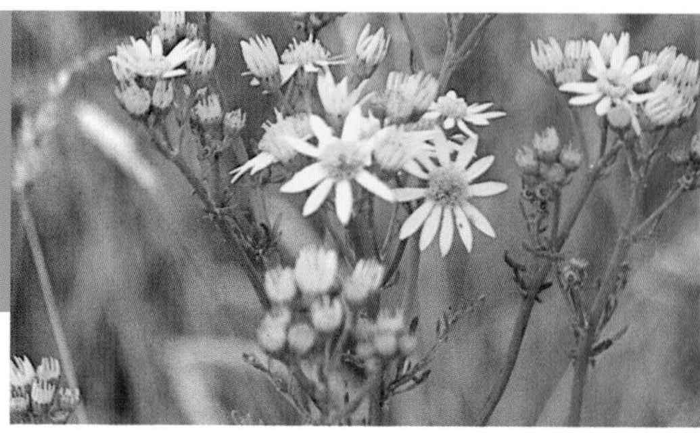

It is best to remove ragwort from any field where horses are kept. Although they rarely eat it, it can have serious health consequences if they do.

Some substances are poisonous to horses in small quantities. Unfortunately, unless an animal is seen ingesting a poison, it is often not possible to tell what caused the problem. Your horse should not have any contact with the common chemical and herbaceous poisons that are listed here. It is also a good safety precaution not to allow him near any ground that has recently been treated with pesticides or herbicides.

Lead

Commonly found in old paint and old car batteries. Ingestion of lead will cause collapse and death. Always ensure that there is no peeling paint in stables.

Plants

It is worth remembering that poison is the plant's defence against being eaten. This is not as much of a problem in deciduous plants as in evergreens. Most evergreen plants are poisonous to some degree. The horse has evolved to eat grasses. Therefore, as a general rule, try to prevent ingestion of large quantities of other herbaceous sources. Some plants, such as St John's wort, are more toxic dry than fresh, and can be very dangerous. Here are the most common poisonous plants and their symptoms.

- Hemlock (*Conium maculatum*). Symptoms include dilated pupils, staggering and, after a few hours, respiratory paralysis.
- Common pokeweed (*Phytolacca americana*). Symptoms include excess salivation because of a burning sensation in the mouth, stomach cramps, vomiting, convulsions, diarrhoea and gastroenteritis.
- St John's wort (*Hypericum perforatum*) and ragwort (*Senecio jacobaea*). Symptoms include loss of appetite, photosensitization (see page 14), convulsions, peeling skin and coma.
- Burweed (*Xanthium strumarium*). Symptoms include lack of appetite and weight loss, depression and a weakened heartbeat.
- Bluebell (*Hyacinthoides non-scripta*). Symptoms include abdominal pain and diarrhoea, skin that feels cold and damp to the touch, vomiting, low temperature and no urination.

Lethal plants

Some of the plants listed above may be lethal if ingested in very large amounts, but the following ones are almost always lethal and you should ensure that there are none anywhere near your horse.

- Yew (*Taxus spp.*)
- Some types of laurel (*Prunus* and *Kalmia spp.*)
- Box (*Buxus sempervirens*)
- Privet (*Ligustrum spp.*)
- Rhododendrons and azaleas (*Rhododendron spp.*)

GRAIN OVERLOAD

Grain can be poisonous if eaten in large quantities. This is called grain overload, and is a potentially life-threatening condition. If left, the grain ferments in the gut, killing off all the friendly micro-organisms. This leads to the release of large quantities of toxin and an imbalance in the normal electrolytes in the horse. Without treatment, this will cause acute diarrhoea, acute laminitis and death. You should always restrict the proportion of grain that your horse gets in his diet.

The vet will use laxatives and absorbents to try to prevent digestion of the grain and speed up its transition through the gut.

Homoeopathy

In the late eighteenth century, Samuel Hahnemann discovered the principle that 'like treats like', which became known as homoeopathy. He found that while large doses of a substance could induce symptoms of a disease, minute, repeatedly distilled preparations of the same substance could be used to treat that disease. Homoeopathy is essentially a form of natural healing: the remedy assists the patient to regain health by stimulating the body's own recovery mechanisms. Its use in domestic animals, including horses, has become more popular with vets and animal owners over the last 20 years or so because of its effectiveness, minimal side effects and lack of drug residues, which is particularly important for competition horses.

There is controversy and debate about the scientific background and the use of homoeopathy, particularly regarding homoeopathic vaccines, but there is little doubt that it can be an effective tool. Homoeopathic remedies come in tablet, powder or liquid form and in various potencies – for example, 3C, 6C, 200C, 1M; these refer to the dilutions of the remedy and, paradoxically, the greater the dilution the more effective the remedy can be.

Using arnica before, during and after a long ride or competition can help prevent bruising and concussion to the feet and legs.

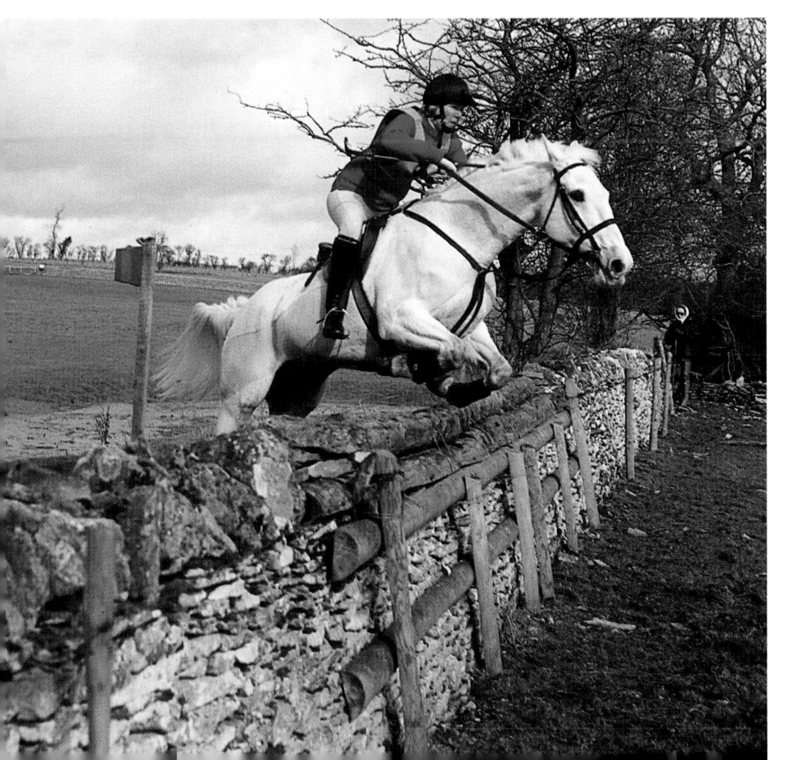

Conditions that can be treated

Conditions where homoeopathic preparations can be effective include the following:

- Sweet itch (see page 23) is an allergic skin condition resulting from the bite of midges. Giving a preparation of an extract of the midge itself daily throughout the season can help prevent and cure the problem.
- Mud fever and rain scald (see page 17) are skin infections of *Dermatophilus congolensis*, which can be treated with Thuja, Arsenicum album or Malindrinum.
- Echinacea is a popular herbal medicine which is used to help boost immunity. Its homoeopathic preparation is used for the same purpose, and also to accelerate wound healing.
- Caulophyllum can be used to assist in labour, and Arnica is used to help prevent and heal bruising and the trauma of foaling.
- To help expel pus from abscesses (see page 26) use low potencies of Hep sulph, and Silica to expel foreign material and repair contaminated wounds – for example, knees grazed on the road.
- For bee stings use Apis mel, and for hives and nettle stings use Urtica urens.
- Long-distance riding can cause bruising to the feet and concussion to the legs. Using Arnica before, during and after the event can help. Ruta grav given earlier in the day can help to prevent the back strain resulting from carrying the rider for several hours.
- Other conditions where homoeopathy has been useful are splints (see page 83), arthritis, laminitis (see page 74), COPD (see page 57), head shaking (see page 91) and colic (see pages 44–45).

Euthanasia

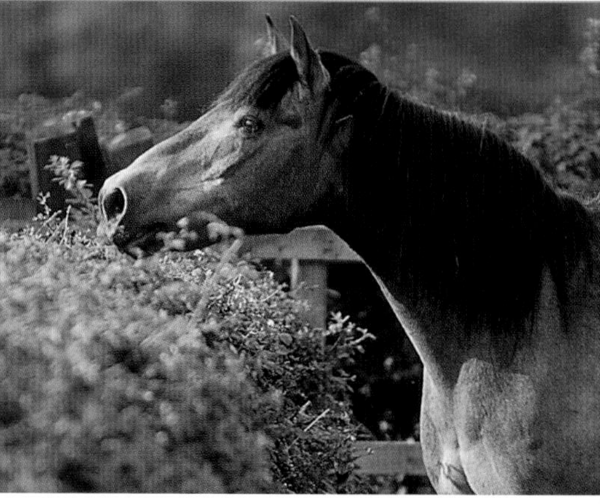

Deciding to let a horse go is one of the hardest decisions to make, but the horse's welfare should always come first.

Euthanasia is probably the hardest decision any horse owner can face. Unfortunately, there are not many horses that pass away in their sleep at night, and this means that the decision regarding quality of life will come down to the owner.

As horses age, obviously they slow down – this is perfectly normal. The difficulty comes in determining whether a horse has a sufficiently good quality of life. An old, stiff horse may not be in pain and if he is bright, alert, in good condition and eating well, it is unlikely that he is suffering. Consulting your vet will help in determining whether a horse is suffering and whether there is further treatment that may help.

It can help to consider beforehand where you would like the euthanasia to occur and what you want to happen to the body, before arranging for the horse to be put down.

Where

A horse is more likely to be calm and relaxed in the familiar surroundings of his home, but it must be possible to move the horse once the euthanasia has occurred. An open area with easy access for vehicles is best.

A horse may only be put down away from home if he is fit to travel – his welfare must come first. The horse may be transported directly to a local veterinary surgery, slaughter house or hunt kennels.

How

Euthanasia can be carried out by either lethal injection or shooting.

A lethal injection involves the overdose of an anaesthetic and this may only be carried out by a veterinary surgeon. A number of different drugs can be used which cause the horse to collapse and become anaesthetized. Once this has occurred, more of the anaesthetic is injected to help stop the heart. This can take up to five minutes. During this time it is common to see rhythmic breathing, and occasional muscle spasms as the muscles relax and react to lower levels of oxygen in the blood system caused by the heart slowing down.

Shooting can be performed by a veterinary surgeon, knackerman, a hunt kennelman, licensed slaughterman or, in an emergency, by an animal welfare inspector, and is normally cheaper than a lethal injection. When a horse is shot, he drops to the ground immediately. Involuntary movement of the legs may accompany this, and there is often significant bleeding from the bullet hole, and from the nose. This is entirely normal, and even if you are prepared for it, can be very distressing to watch.

Disposal

Some slaughterhouses will incinerate horses. This normally incurs a cost, which will usually increase if the horse has been injected or was ill. This is the most common form of disposal, whichever method of euthanasia was used.

Cremation can be carried out only in approved animal crematoria. For an extra fee, it is usually possible to have the ashes returned. There are increasing numbers of rules and regulations concerning burying horses, and this is often not an option.

The death or euthanasia of any animal is never pleasant but decisions are often easier to make if you have already thought about them. It is important always to put the horse's welfare before your own.

Glossary

Analgesic Pain relief, which may be given orally or by injection.

Anti-inflammatory Drug that reduces inflammation.

Antispasmodic Drug that helps to relieve spasm in muscles, especially smooth muscle with respect to colic.

Arrhythmia Any abnormality in the rhythm of the heart.

Arthroscope Form of endoscope (see below) inserted into the joint space to view the inside of the joint.

Ataxia Unsteadiness, lack of co-ordination, often unable to stand.

Autogenous Originating from the patient's own body tissue.

Benign Lump that is not malignant.

Biopsy Removal of a small piece of tissue to facilitate analysis.

Cast Solid bandage, needed to immobilize a limb.

Chondroitin sulphate Simple molecule which has been shown to stimulate replication of joint cartilage and inhibit some of the enzymes that break down cartilage. Its effects have not been 100 per cent proven in the live animal.

Crepitus Crunching felt or heard if a joint is flexed or a fracture moved.

Cryosurgery Use of liquid nitrogen to freeze off (cauterize) lumps or tissue.

Electrocardiogram (ECG) Printout of the electrical currents generated by the heart.

Electrolytes Chemical substances found in the body, whose levels are very dependent on water levels within the body.

Endoscope Form of camera on a long flexible rod, used to view hollow organs or body cavities.

Excision Surgical removal of a piece of tissue.

Glucosamine Simple molecule found in joints and connective tissue, used by the body for cartilage repair. Supplementation may strengthen joints and relieve pain or stiffness. Its effects have not been 100 per cent proven in the live animal.

Granulation tissue New tissue that forms during the repair of a wound. In skin wounds below the knee it may be produced to excess (proud flesh).

Haematoma Blood-filled lump, which can occur in the skin or other organs, commonly caused by trauma. Bruises are a form of haematoma.

Histopathology Examination of tissue sections to determine a disease process.

Hoof testers Pincer-like instrument used to detect and pinpoint solar foot pain.

Hyposodont Tooth of fixed length that continually erupts until it falls out.

Lavage Cleaning of a wound with a liquid.

Lesion Damaged or abnormal tissue.

Ligation Tying of a ligature, used in surgery to constrict tissues such as a blood vessel to prevent bleeding.

Magnetic resonance imaging (MRI) Imaging of soft tissue and bony structures in three dimensions. Not widely available, and at present only large enough to encompass horses' legs.

Malignant Tumour that tends to deteriorate, often spreading to other parts of the same tissue and other tissues in the body. Unless treated, the end result is normally death.

Malocclusion Inability of the teeth to meet in proper alignment.

Mandibular teeth Lower teeth, originating from the mandible.

Maxillary teeth Upper teeth, originating from the maxillar.

Methylsulphonylmethane (MSM) Non-protein source of sulphur with anti-inflammatory properties that are beneficial in the treatment of joint problems, laminitis, respiratory and skin problems.

Opthalmoscope Instrument that magnifies and allows the eye, and back of the eye, to be viewed.

Opthalmology Study of the eyes.

Osteoarthritis Degenerative joint disease.

Palpation Technique of feeling parts of the body by finger touch alone.

Pedunculated Lump that is connected to the body by a stem-like strip of tissue.

Probiotic Oral supplement of the normal bacteria that cover the inside of the digestive tract and aid digestion.

Radiation therapy Treatment of cancerous growths by the use of radiation, in the form of a radioactive injectable substance or topical radioactive wire placed directly over the tumour.

Scintigraphy Imaging of soft tissue and bone after injecting a radioactive isotope into the body, enabling areas of inflammation to be pinpointed.

Secondary infection Infection contracted after an initial viral, bacterial, surgical or traumatic insult. It often occurs through contamination of a surgical site or weakness after an illness.

Spasticity Tightening of muscles, causing stiff or awkward movements.

Systemic treatment Use of oral treatments to attack a specific problem.

Topical treatment External application of a treatment to an affected area.

Tubbing Placing the foot in a warm bucket of water containing salt or Epsom salts, ideally for 5–10 minutes at least twice a day, or as directed by a vet.

Ulcerative Causing ulcers.

Ultrasonography Use of ultrasound to visualize soft-tissue structures and some bony structures.

Unthriftiness General poorness, not doing as well as expected, lack of lustre of coat, general misdemeanour.

Index

Acknowledgements

Executive Editor Trevor Davies
Editor Rachel Lawrence
Executive Art Editor Karen Sawyer
Designer Les Needham
Picture Research Christine Junemann
Production Controller Martin Crowshaw

Photographic Acknowledgements in Source Order

Octopus Publishing Group Limited/
Bob Atkins 12, 28, 36, 37, 41, 47, 52, 62, 64, 85, 86, 91, 97, 99, 101, 108, 124
Houghton's Horses 15, 19, 30, 95, 96
Bob Langrish 4–5, 7, 8, 16, 17, 18, 21, 23, 25, 27, 31, 38 top, 38 centre, 38 bottom, 40, 42, 43, 44, 46, 48, 50, 51, 55, 56, 57, 59, 61, 65, 67, 68, 70, 71, 73, 74, 76, 80, 81, 83, 87, 88, 90, 98, 102, 104, 105, 106, 107, 110, 111, 112, 113, 115 left, 115 right, 116 left, 116 right, 116 centre, 119, 121, 122, 123